BUILDING
THE *Perfect*
STAR

Changing the Trajectory of Sports
and the People In Them

"His ideas and his thoughts and his programs. I really do think that Bob Ward had a lot to do with the all of those winning seasons we had in Dallas. To this day, if you talk to the players he worked with, we are all crazy about him."

Roger Staubach
Dallas Cowboys quarterback, 1969 – 79
Pro Football Hall of Fame

"There is no question he made a tremendous impact on what the NFL did in terms of strength and conditioning. He was way ahead of his time."

Dan Reeves
Dallas Cowboys assistant coach, 1970 – 80
NFL head coach, 1981 – 2003

"Bob Ward introducing martial arts to the sport of football is something I would never have recognized. To me, he is a genius."

Dan Inosanto
Martial Arts trainer and master
One of three students to be trained by Bruce Lee

"Bob Ward is the reason I became an All-Pro. He never stopped coaching. He never stopped teaching. He brought an Eastern European way of thinking to football, and a mental component to the game."

Charlie Waters
Dallas Cowboys safety, 1970 – 78, 1980 – 81
Three-time NFL Pro Bowl

"With Bob Ward, we did things before everybody else did. We were the most physically fit team in the NFL. The improvement in our guys was because of Bob Ward."

Mike Ditka
Dallas Cowboys assistant coach, 1973 – 74, 1975 – 76, 1981
NFL head coach, 1982 – 99
Pro Football Hall of Fame

"Almost everything they are doing now when it comes to training, he was doing it back in the '70s."

Dr. Gene Coleman

Houston Astros strength and conditioning coach, 1976 – 2012

"When I was in college, I wanted to be Bob Ward. Bob was on the forefront in the distinction between coaching someone to hit a golf ball and helping the guy get strong to do what they do better."

Dave Murphy

USC Track and Field, discus and shot

NCAA All-American, 1970

"Dr. Ward was one of the original pioneer researchers to get those of us to understand how performance training goes from theory to the practical and how to take the practical to sport-specific usage. One of the best examples was the work he did with the Dallas Cowboys in the '70s before there was truly a profession."

Brian Weese

Professional trainer, specializing in football player preparation for the NFL Combine

"If you could describe a guru, that's a guru. He is the Swami – not only to tell you what direction to go in terms of lifting weights but what direction in life."

Cliff Harris

Dallas Cowboys safety, 1970 – 79

Cowboys Ring of Honor, 2004

"Bob was an innovator and was just incredible at what he did. Because of his background, and his creativity, and his education, he had this subtle way of saying, 'Let's work some more' without making it feel like you were doing more. He made you want to do it because he made it interesting. He was the epitome of a coach and a comrade."

Bob Breunig

Dallas Cowboys linebacker, 1975 – 84

Three-time NFL Pro Bowler

"What he brought to the NFL was a combination of track, weight lifting, and power lifting. The CrossFit craze that you see today? That is Bob Ward's workout. It's come full circle. This is not new. It's 40 years old, and it originated with Bob Ward."

Butch Johnson
Dallas Cowboys wide receiver, 1976 – 83
Denver Broncos wide receiver, 1984 – 85

"Bob Ward was always looking to do anything he could under the sun. He was a bit out there in that regard. He didn't want to be put in a box for how to get a guy ready to play."

Brian Baldinger
Dallas Cowboys offensive lineman, 1982 – 84; 1986 – 87
Indianapolis Colts, 1988 – 90; Philadelphia Eagles, 1992 – 93
Host and Analyst, NFL Network

BUILDING
THE *Perfect*
STAR

Changing the Trajectory of Sports
and the People In Them

DR. BOB WARD
AND MAC ENGEL
FOREWORD BY RANDY WHITE

Requests for permission should be addressed to: Ascend Books, LLC, Attn: Rights and Permissions Department, 12710 Pflumm Road, Suite 200, Olathe, KS. 66062

10 9 8 7 6 5 4 3 2 1

ISBN: print book 978-0-9961944-3-3
ISBN: e-book 978-0-9961944-4-0

Library of Congress Control Number: 2015947972

Publisher: Bob Snodgrass
Editor: Claire Reagan
Managing Editor: Aaron Cedeño
Publication Coordinator: Christine Drummond
Sales and Marketing: Lenny Cohen and Sandy Hipsh
Dust Jacket and Book Design: Rob Peters

All photos courtesy of Bob Ward unless otherwise indicated.

Every reasonable attempt has been made to determine the ownership of copyright. Please notify the publisher of any erroneous credits or omissions, and corrections will be made to subsequent editions/future printings.

The goal of Ascend Books is to publish quality works. With that goal in mind, we are proud to offer this book to our readers. Please note, however, that the story, experiences, and the words are those of the authors alone.

Printed in the United States of America.

www.ascendbooks.com

CONTENTS

DEDICATION

I dedicate this book to the many giants who have enabled me to have a wonder life. Their guidance brought me a "Many Splendored Career"; those giants pointed me to the principles that enabled me to strive to be "The Best That I Was Meant To Be."

First and foremost, to my family: To Joyce, my amazing wife who has been an invaluable resource for all aspects of my life, my Christian walk, and my career.

Second, to my daughters, their amazing husbands, and their children: Shannon (Mark) Lichty, Erin (Sam) Symmank, my Lichty Grandchildren – Erin – Erik – Scott, and my Symmank Grandchildren – Taylor – Jared – Gabrielle.

Finally, I'd like to pass on "The-Best-That-You-Were-Meant-To-Be Baton" to those who can and must continue to run with it, that they may experience a similar, but unique, wonderful life and career for themselves.

– Bob Ward

• • • •

For Vivian
    Thank you
    I love you
        – Mac Engel

FOREWORD
BY RANDY WHITE

I was a No. 1 draft pick out of the University Maryland in 1975. One of the biggest reasons I was selected that high is because I hit people as hard as I could possibly hit them. Hitting people is what I did, and I did it really well. In my first two seasons in the NFL, I was still playing a position that was foreign to me – linebacker. I was a defensive tackle, but Coach Tom Landry wanted me at linebacker. So I played linebacker and was still good at hitting people.

In my third NFL offseason, in the spring of 1977, Coach Landry moved me back to defensive tackle. There was a difference almost immediately. This was the position I knew, a position where I could hit people more effectively. One day during offseason training, our conditioning coach had us hitting punching bags like a boxer. Predictably, I hit those bags as hard as I possibly

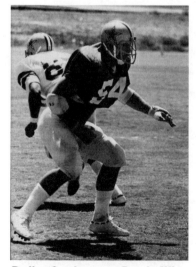

Dallas Cowboys star Randy White was moved to linebacker early in his career before moving back to his normal position of defensive tackle – where he would enjoy a Hall of Fame career.

could. I left a large impression on those heavy bags because I was good at hitting.

Our conditioning coach was Dr. Bob Ward. He looked right at me and said, "The problem is you don't know *how* to hit."

My first thought: *What is this guy telling me, I don't know how to hit?*

Ask anyone who played me if I knew how to hit. Anyone who played me when I was in high school. Anyone who played me when I was in college and won the Outland Trophy *and* the Lombardi Trophy. Or anyone who played me during my first two years in the NFL. They'll all tell you the same thing: I knew how to hit. I was given the nickname "The Manster" for a reason. I was a rookie in 1975, and in my first three years playing for the Dallas Cowboys, I was named to the Pro Bowl, we won the Super Bowl, and I was named co-MVP of the Super Bowl with my friend Harvey Martin – it was the first time two teammates had been named the MVP of a Super Bowl and the first time the award was given to a defensive lineman. I had become a big part of the famous "Doomsday Defense," in part because I was really good at hitting people.

All of those achievements and accomplishments said I knew how to hit. But, when I look back on that third year and what Dr. Ward told me, it was apparent he was right – I did not know *how* to hit. Once I swallowed my ego and my pride, and listened to what he was telling me, then I *really* learned how to hit.

Dr. Bob Ward was revolutionary and saw things in a way most people cannot. He constantly looked to see things in a different light, either for himself or for others. I know he made the Dallas Cowboys a better football team.

Bob had this way of saying you can always get better, you can *always* get better. He could bring you down to earth without making you feel bad or like you failed. He wanted you down to earth because it would keep all of us motivated to be better. Bob was always about improvement and searching for ways to be better in everything. He constantly read books, conducted research, and brought all sorts of new and different ideas and people to the Cowboys in an effort to keep us moving and improving.

When Bob and I were with the Dallas Cowboys in the late '70s, we were one of the best teams in the National Football League. As players, we knew were good, but Bob had this way of creating challenges that pushed all of us even if we didn't want to be or always know we were being pushed. He appealed to our inner sense of curiosity and competitiveness. Never before meeting Bob had I met a guy like him, and the same can be said since our first encounter.

Bob was a true innovator when it came to strength and conditioning as well as nutrition. When I think about Bob, he was really kind of a genius. For those of us who played in the NFL in the '70s and the early '80s, we see Bob Ward everywhere. The man impacted the NFL Combine, the NFL Draft, player analysis and evaluation, workouts, even how a football player takes water breaks.

Bob was foremost a teacher, but he would say to me, "Randy – you don't really teach anybody anything." I pondered on that one for years and years. It really baffled me for a long, long time. He would say, "If you watch a baby in a crib, he does every possible movement you can think of." He explained how a baby twists, turns, rolls, flexes, cries, smiles, laughs, moves his eyes, pulls his ears – a baby does everything. What he was saying was – it's all in there, someone just has to bring it out of you. To be honest, I still really don't get it, but I think I understand it.

Bob would do that a lot, actually. He would say these things that when you first heard them made a lot of sense, then didn't make any sense at all. He said something, you would nod your head like you understood it, and then he would walk away and you'd think, *What the hell is he talking about?* But it would stay with you, whatever he said, and the more you thought about it, what he said was perfectly logical. I never had a strength coach, or really any coach, like him in my entire career.

When I was younger, right out of college and playing football, the reason I liked him so much was because I figured out pretty quick that this guy could make me better. He was the one who pushed me in certain directions. I was his test subject, and I loved it because working with him was so interesting, so much fun, and I knew it was making me a better player. Bob was the one who got me involved in martial arts, in different types of weight lifting, and other exercises that I know made me better. Bob was the one who taught me I didn't know how to hit, and he was right.

I also always liked Bob because he was and is such a good person. The more I got to know him, I realized he's the kind of person who puts so many others before himself. I really think what he did with the Cowboys was his calling. He was meant to do that work, helping make people better at what they were doing, whether it was football or just life. Bob was a big influence on my football career. He helped me achieve the level of success that I attained. More than anything else, Dr. Bob Ward is a great person, and he remains a great friend.

> ***Randy White***
> Dallas Cowboys defensive tackle, 1975 – 88
> Eight-time NFL All-Pro
> Nine NFC Pro Bowl selections
> Super Bowl XII co-MVP
> NFL Defensive Player of the Year, 1978
> Dallas Cowboys Ring of Honor, 1994
> Pro Football Hall of Fame, 1994

PROLOGUE

Dave Murphy badly fumbled in his initial attempts to describe Dr. Bob Ward. It didn't take too long before this picture of masculinity and strength teared up and sounded like he was about to cry. "I don't know why I get emotional when I talk about him," Murphy said. Murphy was an All-American shot putter at USC in the '70s and had worked with Ward both in high school and at Fullerton Community College.

"I know why I do. There are three men in my life who've had an enormous influence on me – one is my dad, another is a friend of the family, and the last one is Bob Ward."

Murphy didn't mean to, or much want to, tear up when talking about a guy whom he had not played for in more than four decades. But he sincerely couldn't help it. When Dave Murphy looked back at the trajectory of his life, he knew that Bob Ward altered it to go to a higher plane. That his life without Bob Ward would not look as good as it does today. He went on to earn his degree from the University of Southern California. He eventually became a teacher and an amateur musician. He's had a good life.

That is Bob Ward's greatest legacy – he changed the trajectory of people, and the trajectory of sports, for the better.

One of America's most established and foremost experts in martial arts – a man named Dan Inosanto – said when he was a freshman at Whitworth College in Spokane, Washington, he idolized Bob Ward, who was a senior at the time. Dan looked up to Bob so much that the subject he chose for his semester term paper in his English class was Bob Ward.

The more people I talked to for this book, the more it dawned on me that the depth and the breadth of this man's life was far greater than a weight room or a football field. The more people I contacted for this book, the more people wanted to talk about Dr. Bob Ward. They wanted to share their stories about this man and the impact he made.

Bob Ward changed the way people looked at a weight room and forced them to see the football field as a giant scientific grid. The brilliance of Bob Ward is both his willingness to listen and his eagerness to continually learn. The man remains, even in his advanced age, the model of old school, traditional values. This is not to say he doesn't have an ego – he does – but he knows enough to know that ultimately he doesn't know very much at all.

Many of the people interviewed for this book said he was a genius. It is true that much of what Ward says and writes is difficult to comprehend, making the material intimidating. At a minimum, they said he was ahead of his time and revolutionary in the field of strength and conditioning and performance enhancement. After reviewing, reading, and poring over studies, stories, and research, it quickly became apparent the impact this man made on pro sports was vast, wide, and relatively unknown. That's the way science is – not many researchers and pioneers are household names. By title, Bob Ward was a conditioning coach. Or maybe even a strength coach. Really, though, he was a scientist.

Bob Ward's fingerprints are all over a great majority of what we see today in the biggest professional sports organization in North America – the National Football League. Someone else would have inevitably introduced the many details he brought to the NFL, but he was the first. People copycat this man to this day without even knowing it.

When it came to strength and conditioning, whatever he tried to pass on or implement with others, he did it himself first. He lifted weights. He played football. He was a coach. He did the research. As one strength and fitness coach said – Bob got in the trenches to see what really worked.

"Bob is the very best combination of what a man in his position should ever have," said Dr. Peter Snell, who won Olympic gold medals in middle distance running for his native New Zealand in the '60s. He later went on to become a doctor and the director of the Human Performance Laboratory at the University of Texas-Southwestern Medical Center in Dallas. "When you take his great practical experiences he had as an athlete and then couple them with his education in exercise and physiology, that is a powerful, powerful combination."

While far from perfect, Bob is an example of clean living. He eats right. He exercises. He never deliberately inflicts stress on himself. This lifestyle explains why the man was such an accomplished decathlete for decades and routinely won amateur track and field events at the highest levels for his age. To see him in his 80s is to see a man who appears to look no older than his mid-60s.

Despite his vast and many achievements professionally, what separates Ward are the differences he made with the many people he worked with for more than four decades. He was respected, loved, and revered as a professional, a husband, a father, and a grandfather.

Some of the most respected men in Ward's era of professional football cite Bob Ward either as the reason for their individual improvement or success, or they credit his presence for why the Dallas Cowboys remained for so long one of the most successful organizations in professional sports.

We all hope to have made a lasting impression. The most visible part of his legacy will likely always be with the Dallas Cowboys and the National Football League, but his real impression is with his family and the people he worked with, from the obscure high school kids in Buena Park, California, to the highly visible pro athletes in Dallas, Texas.

The most we can ask for is to make a difference and for what we did to matter. Bob Ward has done both.

Mac Engel

CHAPTER 1
YOU'RE FIRED

"There's nothing wrong with being fired."
– Ted Turner

Jimmy Johnson's cheeks looked like one of his expensive blowfish that he would pay expensive money to keep in one of his expensive custom-made aquariums. When Jimmy was mad, his face would turn red, his cheeks and jowls turning a deeper shade of crimson. That famous Port Arthur, Texas twang raised a few octaves, and everyone within earshot immediately knew not to screw with him. Jimmy was so mad that his famous hair, hair that seemed not to move even in a tornado, actually fluffed up.

"We're weak!" Jimmy screamed. "We're not strong enough!"

The guy sitting across his desk at the Dallas Cowboys headquarters in Irving, Texas, was not some obscure equipment guy or low-level intern who would look at the floor and merely nod in fear. The guy Jimmy was screaming at was one of the most revered, revolutionary, and respected men in his field. He was a 57-year-old man whose ideas, concepts, research, and application transformed the NFL, sports, and strength training. He was also built like a Sherman tank. Jimmy didn't care who he was or the fact that in fighting terms this man could easily have turned him into a pile of broken bones. Jimmy had just told this man that his team was weak, not strong enough. Jimmy had just told Dr. Bob Ward he was bad at his job.

Few men were more accomplished in his field at creating new ways to maximize performance than Bob Ward, but in this moment, none of that mattered. Few men were any better at trying to create the slightest edge, but in this moment, that was irrelevant.

Ward was and is a kind, good-humored man, but there was no way he was going to take this type of scathing performance review from anybody up to and including his boss, the head coach of the Dallas Cowboys. Ward looked across at Jimmy. Rather than cower in agreement with a "Sorry, I'll do better next time, Coach," he simply stated, "Show me the ocular evidence."

He may as well have said, "Go to hell."

Jimmy did not appreciate Ward's ode to Shakespeare's *Othello* with that "ocular proof" line. Ward was being a wise ass, something he was quite good at since the time he was a kid growing up in less than ideal conditions near Los Angeles. Ward was not the type of man to raise his voice or yell at anyone, but he could deliver a one-liner.

This meeting took place in the early part of 1990. Here was one of the most respected men in his job squaring off with the brash new head coach of the Dallas Cowboys, desperate to prove he was worthy of replacing the legend – Coach Tom Landry. Depending on the view, both men were right, yet neither was going to move a fraction from their stance.

Both men realized that to return this franchise to its previous standing in American sports would require the boldest of actions, or as Ward would say, they needed to cut the Gordian Knot. The Dallas Cowboys had a problem because, at that time, they were terrible. Jimmy knew it. Bob knew it. They both knew to make them better would require something drastic.

To Jimmy, the Cowboys *were* weak. To Ward, the Cowboys were strong. Jimmy was right, and so was Ward. Ward also knew he would lose this argument, and ultimately a job he loved.

The Cowboys had just completed their first season under Jimmy, finishing as the worst team in the National Football League with a 1 – 15 record. The last time before 1989 the Dallas Cowboys had been the worst team in the NFL was 1960, their first year of existence. The 1989 Dallas Cowboys were historically awful. The next closest God-awful team in 1989 was the Atlanta Falcons, finishing with an enviable three wins. Jimmy knew his team was bad, and the last thing he wanted was an argument of any sort about the specifics of a miserable year. What Ward wanted to show his head coach was a giant stack of computer printouts that analyzed every player from that 1989 team, a great many of whom were indeed quite strong.

To Jimmy, there was no point in reviewing all of these "analytics" – which in 1990 was not the commonly-used word in sports that it would become 20 years later – that Ward had tracked and categorized about a bunch of players the head coach was aiming to dump the first chance he got. Jimmy did not care about analysis. In that moment, had Ward presented Jimmy a check for $10 million, Jimmy may well have responded with the same eruption.

"Jimmy wanted a more conventional guy in that job. He wanted a basic strength and conditioning program," Ward recalls. "I did not want to be relegated to only that. I knew I had much more to offer than that."

Jimmy wanted a strength coach who would pump iron and make his guys "jacked." Ward could do that, but his expertise went considerably beyond the weight room. He earned a doctorate from Indiana University for reasons beyond a bench press. In his mind, the problem of the 1989 Dallas Cowboys was not one of strength. That was too easy. That was too simple. That was also not accurate.

"If you need 400 pounds of bench press strength, why lift more than that?" Ward asks. "There are plenty of greenhorn coaches who say, 'We're going to work, and we're going to work, and we're going to work some more.' But I think what you have to do is allow for a little recovery, growth, and restoration. I think that's what happened to us [that 1989 season]. We worked harder than ever in training camp, but we just reached a state of exhaustion. You cannot gain super adaptation levels when you're tired. It's just impossible."

If it were merely about strength, the Dallas Cowboys were fine. In terms of strength, the 1989 Cowboys were one of the better teams in the National Football League. The problem was they were not good enough, and no amount of weight lifting was going to change that reality. As history would later prove, Jimmy Johnson was no dummy, but he also came from the era of coaches who believed more was not only better, it was essential to success. His training camps for the Dallas Cowboys at St. Edwards University in Austin were renowned for their brutality. Cowboys Pro Bowl fullback Daryl "Moose" Johnston once said of a Jimmy training camp: "I come to camp in the best shape of my life. Six weeks later, I'm totally beaten up and in the worst shape of my life, so it takes the first month of the regular season to get back into top condition."

Ward had been the conditioning coach of the Cowboys since 1976, and he knew a good football team from a bad one. He had played football in high school and college, and he was not blind, or deaf, or dumb. He knew talent and God-given ability. Ward was one of the few people Jimmy retained on his staff from the Tom Landry regime after Jerry Jones bought the franchise in February of that year. Tom was a God in professional football, and Jerry Jones firing him after he bought the team would make him a villain to loyal fans of this franchise forever, regardless of any future success the team may, and did, have. That reality weighed on Jimmy, something that even in the heat of their confrontation after the season was not lost on Ward.

During the early portion of that first season, after yet another loss, Johnson and Ward were heading into a large dinner with the staff. "Just gimme' a chance," Johnson said. "Stay with me." It was still early yet in that season, and Johnson needed allies to buy what he was selling. As the season progressed, he made moves indicating he was no longer worried about allies but just wins – moves signaling he was going to do it *his* way.

Jimmy had decided to completely tear the team down, and during that 1989 season, it became apparent to Ward he was not going to last too long in this job. Johnson and Jones traded running back Herschel Walker to the Minnesota Vikings. This Walker trade would later become a verb in the NFL, and the many parts of the trade became essential to the Dallas Cowboys' three '90s Super Bowl wins.

It was unusual that Ward had managed to remain in this job after Jimmy took over the team. Most coaches assemble staffs of people they either know, or those who come recommended to them by people they trust. Jimmy had been in the college game and had tremendous success at the University of Miami where he won multiple national titles; he produced a long list of NFL stars, like Reggie White, Vinny Testaverde, Michael Irvin, and on, and on. Jimmy knew plenty of strength and conditioning coaches who could fill Ward's job. Ward had an impressive resume (and a contract), so Johnson gave him a chance, although in retrospect it was more of a half-hearted opportunity.

Strength and conditioning coaches are usually their own entities in a sports franchise and operate not necessarily on the fringe, but often have more latitude than other coaches on the team. "I was a sports scientist who happened to be in control of conditioning, at least when Coach Landry's regime was in," Ward reflects. "When Jimmy came in, I was no longer in charge of a total conditioning program."

After a first season that was so bad, there was no way a head coach was not going to change everything up to and possibly including the paint color of the building. In this moment though, when Jimmy said the Cowboys were weak, Ward took exception. There was strength, and then there was *strength*. This is not semantics. The Cowboys' problem was not simply that of weight lifting, of bicep curls, lunges, squats, or any other exercise in a weight room. There was strength in a weight room, and *strength* on the field. You can have one without the other. The New York Giants had both.

Ward would prove to Jimmy this was not about your basic off and on the field strength, for the latter of which he was accountable. He had the anecdotal, and ocular, proof they were strong and not good enough.

• • • •

The Meadowlands in New Jersey in December can be miserable. It can be a bitterly cold place. The wind swirls and can cut your bones like a handsaw. The AstroTurf at old Giants Stadium was about as soft as a driveway. This place was palatable only if you were winning. By the time the Cowboys came out of the tunnel onto the field at Giants Stadium for the rare Saturday game on December 16, 1989, they were not winning anything, and now they were cold. The temperature at kickoff for the Cowboys and Giants was 20 degrees. With the breeze blowing in from the Northwest, it was a balmy 7 degrees below zero.

The first year of the Jerry Jones/Jimmy Johnson era was an embarrassment. By this point, they'd already won the one game they would for the entire season. Although the team had finished the preseason 3-1, since that moment, it looked like the whole thing would sink under the hubris of two arrogant men who had no idea how success in the oil and gas industry (Jerry) or at the University of Miami (Jimmy) would translate into the cutthroat world of professional football. Things would eventually come around, but not in this first season and not on this particularly nasty December afternoon.

The Giants were good, and this was one of the better teams head coach Bill Parcells had during his eight-year tenure in New York. Before kickoff during warm-ups on the field, Parcells openly discussed with his quarterback, Phil Simms, the desire to finish this game in under three hours. He knew his team was markedly better. He had a famous football roster, after all, with names such as Lawrence Taylor, Phil Simms, Carl Banks, OJ Anderson, Bart Oates, Terry Kinard, Pepper Johnson, Leonard

Marshall, Mark Ingram, and a bunch of other guys who'd won Super Bowls. In professional football, this team remains synonymous with power, manhood, and strength. Former Cowboys guard Nate Newton said playing against this Parcells' team was hard because "they were *men*" – by "men" he meant they were men who could kick your ass.

In this game, the Giants were kicking the Cowboys' ass. There was one sequence that confirmed to Ward everything he needed to know about that entire team, and that while they were strong in a weight room, ultimately, they were weak and simply not good enough on the field.

The Giants led 15-0 to start the fourth quarter, and the Cowboys had the ball at the 1-yard line. It was first down, so they would have a total of four chances to advance the ball 36 inches to score a touchdown. They were likely not going to win the game, but at least they would avoid a shutout and have something to feel good about from this otherwise miserable afternoon. At least they would score a touchdown against *this* defense. At least they could show they hadn't quit or given up in a game that was essentially over and a season that was long gone. Things didn't play out the way they had hoped; the result was neither surprising nor pretty.

- On first down, Cowboys running back Paul Palmer was stopped by linebacker Pepper Johnson for no gain.

- On second down, fullback Broderick Sargent was stopped by Carl Banks and Pepper Johnson for no gain.

- On third down, Cowboys rookie quarterback Troy Aikman's pass was caught by tight end Steve Folsom for a touchdown. The Cowboys had scored the touchdown. But, on further review by the officials, the play was overturned. Folsom's knee had touched the ground before the goal line. There was no touchdown. The Cowboys had one more shot, and rather than settle for a weak field goal, Jimmy went for it. Sitting up in his normal spot in the coaches' box at the top of Giants Stadium, however, Ward was prepared for the Cowboys to be stopped on fourth down.

- On 4th-and-1 from inside the 1, Paul Palmer was stopped for a three-yard loss by Carl Banks and a fleet of other Giants. The Meadowlands erupted, and America's Team meekly headed to its own bench, its damaged pride further eroded and its confidence shot to hell.

The Cowboys could not advance the ball 36 inches for a touchdown. 36 inches.

"That was the whole thing right there," Ward remembers. "It wasn't because we weren't strong enough. We lacked the situational techniques."

The game ended in two hours and 44 minutes, but it felt more like 10 hours and 88 minutes. The Cowboys lost 15-0. The entire season had been like this – other teams gleefully punishing the Cowboys after more than two decades of having it handed to them by America's Team. This was about revenge, and in this case, there was but one grave. The Cowboys had gained only seven first downs against the Giants and finished with 108 total yards. In professional football, these numbers are about as bad as it gets.

Looking back, Ward says, "All of those years, we beat everybody up in the NFL. In that one year, everybody could not wait to beat the Dallas Cowboys…It was awful."

After the game, Parcells walked over to Troy Aikman on the field. Aikman had been the first overall pick in the 1989 NFL Draft, and his rookie season was effectively a hazing session by other teams. In this game, he had been terrorized and beaten into the ground all game by the Giants defense. Parcells told Aikman a day like this was going to serve him well in the future. That this would ultimately make him stronger, which Ward realized, too. Parcells knew as bad as the Cowboys were at that moment, they were going to be just as good.

As is customary, after the game, the team immediately boarded a chartered plane in New Jersey to return to Dallas. As is not customary, when the team bus returned to team headquarters, the coaches did not go home. Jimmy Johnson pulled the coaching staff off the bus and called a staff meeting; he was still livid about the team's inability to score a touchdown from 1-yard out with four tries. In his mind, the reason was simple: This team was weak.

On this team that could not move a ball 36 inches was a roster featuring Aikman, Michael Irvin, Kevin Gogan, Daryl "Moose" Johnston, Ken Norton, Mark Tuinei, Mark Stepnoski, and Nate Newton. All of these players would become integral pieces of a team that would later become an NFL dynasty and the model of strength and intimidation. Four of the players – Tuinei, Newton, Stepnoski, Johnston – were already strong, but in a moment when they needed to gain but one yard, they were overpowered by strength.

"We may be as big as [other teams], but we're not as strong, as physical as they are and that was obvious down in that goal line," Jimmy Johnson said a few days later. "We are a not a physical football team."

Anybody can learn to lift a lot of weight. Not everybody knows how to be physical. There is a big difference between strong and physical. Bob knew that. So did Jimmy.

• • • •

More than a month later, the season mercifully over, Jimmy Johnson blew up at his strength coach when he responded to the claim that the Cowboys were "not strong enough."

When Ward responded with the retort, "Give me the ocular proof," Jimmy snapped.

"I could find a hundred guys to replace you!" he screamed.

It was a threat, but Ward also knew Jimmy was correct. Despite Ward's extensive experience, his vision, and his knowledge, in the mind of a new head coach, his position was expendable and easily replaced.

A strength and conditioning job in the NFL is in high demand, and Jimmy could have easily found more than 100 qualified candidates to replace Ward with but one phone call. The irony is that a few years later, it was Jerry Jones who uttered the phrase, "500 coaches could coach the Dallas Cowboys and win a Super bowl," that later proved prophetic. He replaced Jimmy with Barry Switzer who won the final of the Cowboys' three '90s Super Bowl victories.

Ward knew the Cowboys' issues weren't merely about strength, the Cowboys were indeed strong. To prove his point, Ward had called the strength coach of the New York Giants, Johnny Parker, to get the maximum bench press figures of each of the starting defensive front six players – the guys who had stopped the Cowboys from gaining one yard, 36 inches back on December 16, 1989. The front six players ultimately make the biggest impact on whether an opposing team can move a ball in short, compact areas where collisions are severe and space is ferociously earned. Ward matched up the bench press figures of the players who directly collided in that ill-fated sequence.

Cowboy, Position, Best Bench Press	NY Giant, Position, Best Bench Press
Mark Tuinei, Left tackle, 485	*Leonard Marshall, Right end, 405*
Nate Newton, Left guard, 500	*Erik Howard, Nose tackle, 475*
Mark Stepnoski, Center, 470	*John Washington, Left end, 375*
Crawford Ker, Right guard, 535	*Lawrence Taylor, Linebacker, 315*
Jeff Zimmerman, Right tackle, 450	*Pepper Johnson, Linebacker, 365*
Steve Folsom, Tight end, 405	*Carl Banks, Linebacker, 300*
Cowboys bench press average: 474 pounds	**Giants bench press average: 365 pounds**

The Cowboys problem was clearly not the weight room. Ward believed and had preached that strength is not about the weight room, a best bench, or how many reps you can complete. Ward still believes real strength is total, "Every component is involved in human performance. Strength alone is not enough." Although the Cowboys were strong, they lacked that trifecta of strength – mental, physical, emotional.

He had been in the NFL for 14 seasons, and he was well-versed in that "what the head coach wanted, the head coach was going to get" mentality. Bob knew he was not Jimmy's guy, which was usually enough for a dismissal. He also knew that his contract had expired.

After their blowup, Jimmy approached Bob with a proposal allowing him to ease out of the job as a bridge to finding a different opportunity. Jimmy did not want to fire a man who had been with the organization for so long and had been so important to so many in sports. But Bob didn't give him any choice.

"Jimmy – just go ahead and fire me," was all he said.

After a brief pause, Jimmy replied, "You're fired."

Ward accepted that it was Jimmy's team and he had the right to hire the guy he wanted for that position. This was the end. Like most careers in professional sports, there was no parade, or ceremony. They just end, often abruptly, and with a great deal of sadness and confusion at home.

When Ward left the Dallas Cowboys in the early part of 1990, it was a low point in a professional existence that, to that point, had been a steady ascension. Leaving these jobs is exceptionally difficult; the position unknowingly becomes an enormous part of a person's identity, status, and social structure. There is a pride and an ego-boost to being affiliated with the Dallas Cowboys, or any professional sports team for that matter.

"When I left, I had mixed emotions," Ward recollects. "On the one hand, I really was sad to leave the Dallas Cowboys. The coaching, the players, the friends I had made, the staff. There is a prestige that comes with a job like that.

"On the other hand, I was relieved, too. Jimmy's perception of my job and vision of it were different. With Tom Landry, I had been allowed to work not only on strength and conditioning of all of the players on the team, but I'd been allowed to explore new methods and ideas that would broaden their conditioning and keep them motivated. Landry allowed me to compile data on the players and do research that would enable us to find and do the elements that would improve player performance, and player selection."

Even against the New York Giants, had the Cowboys scored that precious touchdown, advancing a ball an additional 36 inches across a white line was not going to save Ward's job. It didn't matter what his credentials were.

In that moment, to one man trying to prove that he knew what he was doing, Ward was simply in the way. He was expendable.

Neither Jimmy Johnson nor Dr. Bob Ward could have realized that more than 20 years later both men would leave a footprint wide and eternal on sports, and more specifically on the NFL. Jimmy is credited as the architect of the '90s dynasty Dallas Cowboys while Ward is cited as the strength and conditioning pioneer who revolutionized training for the game.

"Bob was ahead of everybody. I mean, *everybody*," said Texas Rangers strength and conditioning consultant Dr. Gene Coleman, who served in the same job for the Houston Astros from 1978 to 2012. "He was doing these things before anybody else. Everything we are doing today [in sports], Bob was doing them in the '70s and '80s."

Ward did not have the capability of making an athlete more than what he was; he could not take a piece of $3 fried chicken and turn it into $75 steak. Ward could not make that 1989 Cowboys offensive line physical, or any more than what they were, which in that moment was not good enough.

As Ward often says, the genetic code determines most of us, but the remainder is a fiercely competitive area that can be affected, and improved. Once the genetic code is determined, the rest is up to us.

So much of what Ward taught in the '70s and '80s, much of which was later discarded, has come back and even been expanded upon in 2015.

Many staples in the NFL and in sports today from computer analysis – i.e. "analytics" – extensive player analysis and evaluation, hydration, rest, speed explosion, over training, martial arts, CrossFit, and NFL Combine preparation, Ward had a hand in creating, implementing, developing, and enhancing.

Ward recognized the limits to his position, but he also knew there was a way to make what you have better in anything. That there are methods to maximize your code's potential. There are ways to maximize your chances to get those 36 inches, to give yourself the best chances of succeeding and winning in the never-ending competition that is life.

The first thing you have to do is figure out what the code is, where you are ideally suited, and then how to get where you decide you are headed. That's not endemic to sports. That's life. There have been few people in the history of the National Football League who were and are any better, or more inventive, at doing this than Bob Ward.

"Bob Ward changed the game forever from a strength and a conditioning standpoint," said former Dallas Cowboys quarterback Danny White, who was with the team from 1976 to 1988. "It wasn't just working on the arms or the legs or the conditioning, it was about the soul and spirit. Bob Ward in my opinion was the most underrated part of the Dallas Cowboys' dynasty in the '70s and the '80s. The guy who had more of an impact than any other person in the Cowboys organization other than Coach Tom Landry was Dr. Bob Ward."

Ward's Words
Jimmy Johnson and Practicing Success

In my one year with Jimmy Johnson, 1989, I saw quickly he was nothing like Tom Landry. Jimmy was fiery, and he would yell and scream. After a game, Coach Landry would really not say too much, but Jimmy would.

We started that first season under Jimmy 0-8. We were really bad. Everybody was beating us. On November 5, we went to play the Washington Redskins, our big rival. The Redskins were pretty good that year, and at the time our No. 1 draft pick, quarterback Troy Aikman, was hurt. We had Steve Walsh as the quarterback.

We had the lead for the second time all season at the half. We were leading by seven in the fourth quarter; with four minutes remaining in the game, Roger Ruzek kicked a 43-yard field goal to put us up by 10 points. We won the game 13-3. It was our only win of the year.

In the locker room after the game, all of the guys were excited, and you could tell what a relief it was. It had been such a long season, and it was only half way over. Jimmy Johnson had Roger Ruzek – in the middle of the locker room – re-enact that fourth-quarter field goal. The whole thing, like Charlie Brown and Lucy. It was just pretend, but Jimmy as the deep snapper, the holder, and Ruzek both go through the field goal like they were doing it again.

I had never seen anything like that before.

CHAPTER 2

A DIFFICULT START

"How do we learn most effectively? Pain and Pleasure."
– Dr. Bob Ward

In reviewing the genetic code for Robert Daryl Ward, fighting for the extra 36 inches that he built a career around should never have factored into the equation. In reviewing his genetic code, an extra 36 inches should never have mattered.

Bob Ward should have been a drunken disaster who ended up living under a bridge. He built himself up from damn close to nothing. From what Ward grew up with and around, his adult life should have been another American tragedy; he should be another sad statistic, not the slice of Americana we want to believe is possible through hard work and determination. How Ward arrived at being one of the most instrumental men in his field is a testament to the power of perseverance as well as to both his mother and his grandmother.

He was born in Huntington Park, California, on July 4, 1933 – he was unofficially a part of the "in between" generation, after World War I but before World War II. He saw and experienced first-hand the crippling effects of the Great Depression that paralyzed America until the start of WWII. Ward was born right in the middle of it.

By the timeline, Ward is actually a member of "The Greatest Generation." They had their problems, but what separates that era is the millions of self-starting Americans who saw and created opportunities and continually moved forward. When former U.S. President Ronald Reagan painted his America, this is the era he recalled so fondly. They came right out of the Depression, won a war, and went on to redefine a nation.

Ward was the fourth of six children born to a German mother who was iron tough and a father he barely knew. His father fought for the United States Army in WWI and was exposed to the brutally hellish conditions on the Western Front in France; he survived the war, but like so many Americans and fighting soldiers who returned to their respective homes, he was forever changed. Ward later learned that his dad was in an area where the German military forces used the infamous mustard gas – which normally affected the skin, eyes, and other exterior areas. There's no way to know the type of psychological impact that experience, as well as many other horrors, left on his father. By the time Ward was a kid, his dad was a mess, an alcoholic, and not around much.

Ward was much too young to understand that his father was likely battling the effects of what is now widely accepted as Post Traumatic Stress Disorder. He just knew his dad worked and his dad drank.

Before Ward was born, and after WWI, his parents had their first two children. The oldest, a girl named Lorraine, died in a gas furnace accident. The second oldest, a boy named Albert, was accidentally injured by hot steam while experiencing a seizure and subsequently died from his injuries.

Ward could never fully understand the effects these tragedies had on his parents or know if these events led to his father's plunge into a bottle of booze.

His parents eventually separated when he was a kid, but the load on his mom was too much. She needed help, so she put her four remaining children – Marilyn, Bob, Maury (Maurice), and Paul – in a home. It was not quite an orphanage, but not quite a Boys and Girls Club, either; it was called The Boys' and Girls' Aid Society. The kids who came to such places were often castoffs from parents who could not handle their parental responsibility. From 1939 to 1941, Ward and his brothers and sister lived there, a time that no doubt left a deep impression in the early developmental years of all of their lives.

Despite his outward toughness, Ward was still just six years old when his mom dropped him and his siblings off at the center. "You had to be tough," Ward says looking back. "You had to fight with the kids. I learned a lot.

"Mom would visit every once in a while. It made me sad. Imagine a young kid and how they would respond psychologically. I would tough it out, but then she would come and that's when I'd get really emotional. When she left, I would sit on the curb and cry like a little baby."

The children were segregated by age and gender, so he did not have the chance to see his brothers and sister on a regular basis. Every so often, they would all be allowed to stay in the same room together, usually when their mother would come to visit. Many times, Bob would chase her car when she drove away.

"I remember cryin' a lot when my mother would leave us there."

Ward lived in a dorm that featured a large hall with beds set up, military style. The kids would routinely jump from bed to bed to bed, raising hell the way little boys often do. There was not a lot of time, however, for this spontaneous kid fun. This was decades before the time when youth sports adopted, some might argue stupidly, a year-round schedule for baseball, softball, basketball, soccer, and even football. Back then, kids played all sports, and at the home, he did it all. He learned gymnastics there, how to pole vault, and something that he feels was essential to his life's work – movement. Bob Ward was horrible at sitting still. He remains horrible at sitting still to this day but has since been able to channel that hyperactivity.

Life in these aid centers was organized with jobs, chores, crafts, education, and sports. There was praise, there was work, and there was punishment. Kids who screwed up were put in "the box"; this was not some prison-style solitary confinement, rather merely a name on a board and a means to take away privileges, such as playing games and other activities. Bob Ward's name was not a frequent visitor to "the box" because, despite the problems at home that led him to this place, he did know right and wrong. He knew where the line was, not that he didn't cross over it from time to time. He also, as Jimmy Johnson later learned, had a quick tongue. Bob was a wise ass, even as a boy. His mouth, however, was not an attempt at belligerence; he'd throw a one-liner to make someone laugh and as a deflection from something going on much deeper.

His mother eventually took her children out of the home to live with her and their father, but that "reconciled" relationship was doomed. His parents simply could not get along, so another separation happened, this time permanently. "I do remember when I was 6 and mom and dad were screaming and yelling at each other," Ward said. "Dad was drunk. I can recall seeing my dad hit my mother. She was a tough gal, too."

They were living in a small home not too far from Hollywood, but closer to what is now Bob Hope Airport in Burbank, California. The parenting role was a bad fit for Ward's father. When his parents separated for good, his dad bolted to Albuquerque and eventually to Nevada, leaving the four kids behind. Child support payments were virtually non-existent.

The last time Ward saw his father was when he was 10. Maybe he was 12. "You don't think that left an impression on me?" Ward asks rhetorically. "Are you kidding me?"

Ward is not sure when his father died. He thinks he died in his early-60s while living in Las Vegas. Ward made no attempt to attend his father's funeral.

His mother would marry three more times, and Ward had but one decent relationship with one of those men. The next man she married was older – Bob figured she did so because he had some money; those two had some type of relationship. After he died, his mother married twice more to men Ward describes as "drunks."

His mother was a florist for a while, but she really made her way working the factory lines at the local Lockheed plant. The lines she worked produced airplanes the United States military used in World War II. Ward also lived with his grandmother and a grandfather who was blind during this time. It was "Grannie" – a second generation American – who was the stabilizing pillar for the family.

One evening when Bob was a kid in the early '40s, the Ward family was in the living room listening to the radio when Ward's second stepfather, who had been drinking, turned belligerent toward the kids after he told them he wanted to listen to a different radio station. Grannie told him to "Get out of here!" and he ran out the door and down the street.

Ward remembers, "We followed him out the door yelling at him. He grew angry and turned around and came running back with what appeared to be the intent to hit us."

That's when Grannie came out with her broom and hit him so hard it gave him a black eye. His step-dad then ran back out of the house, Grannie chasing him out with the broom screaming, "Don't you come back!" This was not the norm every night for the Wards, but it was not exactly uncommon.

They did not starve and were not flush with money, but they did have their share of noise, dysfunction, and drama.

A few years later, after moving out of his grandparents' house, his mother rented a garage apartment to a strapping ex-serviceman with whom Ward once did construction jobs around Los Angeles. Ward, then a teenager, would step into the truck and the first thing that guy did was to hit the hard stuff – whiskey, usually. All of this negative exposure to booze basically deterred Ward away from recreational drugs and alcohol. He experimented a little with whiskey and whatever else in high school because that's what a high school kid does, but he never developed a taste – or need – for it like the many other male "role models" in his life had.

"I do remember coming home after I'd had a little whiskey," he admits. "The room was just spinning and spinning. But that was it, no more."

Bob has never been angry or bitter about his home, or the lack of a reliable father figure. It's what it was. He forgave all of them. Ward is like every other member of that generation – you dealt with it, you didn't bitch, and you moved on. All of that dysfunction did leave a bruise and scars, of course. "What we experience in our lives is never forgotten. I do believe that because it's based on pretty good science," he reflects. "You might suppress things over time, but as you lose your toughness, those insecurities start to come forth."

But all of that dysfunction also helped create a man who was independent, and quietly, his persona embraced the description of the title of a popular TV show that began in 1949 – *The Lone Ranger*.

Bob Ward had plenty of reasons as a kid to be a delinquent, a punk, or even a high school drop out, plenty of reasons to stop, give up, or follow the lead of his absent father. Whenever Ward went looking for a dad, they were gone, drunk, or non-existent. Eventually, rather than go on another fruitless journey for a dad, Ward just stopped looking. As simple as it sounds, he figures his involvement in the Cub Scouts, Boy Scouts, and a local church provided him with a role model to follow: "That's who my fathers were – the 'Scouts."

The Cub Scout Promise reads: "I, [name], promise to do my best, To do my duty to God and my country, To help other people, and To obey the law of the Pack." A good code to live by as far as Ward was concerned.

While he was in the Scouts, America was knee-deep in World War II. This was a time the Wards were living in Burbank, not too far from the Pacific Ocean and Hollywood, but much closer to the factory that produced long-range bomber planes that flew missions in Japan. In fact, Bob would watch these planes on the street in front of his house being towed from the factory to the airport.

There were air raid wardens, ration cards, and the Lockheed factory had a camouflage net with fake homes to hide the building. Patriotism was at an all-time high, and a young boy was susceptible to movies, the power of Uncle Sam's propaganda, and the lure of a green and white painted military jeep. When Ward was a little boy, local army bases would routinely send some young recruits down to the elementary schools in GI jeeps to give the kids rides. Ward would eagerly hop in the jeep and, with adulation in his eyes for the Marines up front, would happily bounce around in the back as it jumped curbs and took corners a bit too fast.

Ward grew up in a region of Southern California that was heavily influenced by World War II and Hollywood's rapidly expanding footprint on American culture. Not too far down from Ward's Burbank home was the venerable Rose Bowl Stadium in Pasadena, which was just down the road from The Boys' and Girls' Aid Society. In 1942, the game was moved from the Rose Bowl to Duke Stadium in North Carolina for fear of attack from Japanese forces, which had attacked Pearl Harbor in Hawaii just the previous month. It is the only time in the Rose Bowl's history that the game was not played at the Rose Bowl Stadium, and Ward noticed. Like so many of his generation, America mattered to Bob Ward; to him, "God and Country" was not merely a disposable slogan of a "Buy America" bonds drive.

• • • •

Whatever dysfunction existed at home was reason enough for Ward to keep running around. He didn't want to go home, so he stayed active.

He was a good – not great – athlete and a C student. There were different paths Ward could walk, but he fell into sports because he was good at them and liked playing them. They were his passion. For a man who made his life's work education and teaching, there is little trace of it during his time at Burbank High School, other than that he gravitated toward sports and a weight room that was in its infancy.

He was also good at football, and he was on a good team. One of his teammates was Paul Cameron, who later would play running back at UCLA. In his senior year at UCLA, Cameron finished third in the voting for the Heisman Trophy. He was drafted by the Pittsburgh Steelers where he played one season and had seven interceptions in 1954. Cameron finished his career for the BC Lions of the Canadian Football League (CFL) where he was an All-Star.

Ward was not as good as Paul Cameron, but he was a starter. He was also equally adept at screwing around and being a wise ass.

"I jacked around way too much," he recalls. "I wasn't dumb, I just wasn't serious. I'm sorry I did it. It hampered my ability later on. It really did. The early years are critical to maximum genetic development. There is substantial research to indicate that if you don't learn 'Fundamental Skills' early, like by 12 years old, you never achieve maximal genetic potential."

Ward would later go on to earn a Master's Degree at the University of Washington and his Doctor of Physical Education (PED) in Biomechanics from Indiana University, yet one of his biggest regrets is that he did not take school seriously enough when he was a kid.

Around the time he was a teenager in Burbank, and not too far from Ward's house, sat Venice Beach in Santa Monica, just north of downtown Los Angeles. Now, it's a tourist attraction, but in the '30s and '40s, it was an epicenter of activity, of movement and exercise. Ward became one of the early members to use Venice Beach's internationally famous "Muscle Beach" as a place to move, exercise, and get in shape. He began to hang out there in the late '40s.

There is some debate about who started Muscle Beach, but in the beginning – in the '30s – it was a tumbling mat, a piece of carpet. The area was set up a few hundred yards south of the Santa Monica Pier, just off the ocean. Back then, Muscle Beach consisted mostly of just gymnastics equipment, and it was free. At a time when nobody had money, Muscle Beach was something to do, a sight to see. People would go there to watch the gymnasts work on their tumbling skills or their flights in the air. Returning soldiers from World War II would congregate there to work out as well.

Bob Ward's high school picture, taken for his senior year at Burbank High School in 1951.

"There was no working out the way we think today of people working out," Ward explains. "It was a whole potpourri of people doing gymnastics. I can remember guys doing flips off swings and double flips. It was just incredible to watch all of this in the sand and the beach. These guys were all in fantastic shape. These guys were crazy daredevils."

What happened on Venice Beach would transform damn near everything involved in sports. Muscle Beach was completely counter to the ideas and concepts that Ward was hearing from his high school coaches – beliefs which were widely held at the time.

"Bob – you don't want to just build muscles up," his Burbank High School football coaches told him.

"Most of the coaches of that time all told us 'Muscle Heads' that – 'You're going to get muscle bound when you have to be able to catch the ball,'" Ward says.

Ward was well into his teenage years when he started playing around with weight lifting; his body's improvement had a definite impact on his self-esteem. The more he lifted, the bigger his muscles grew, the better he felt. He eventually began to play around with the core fundamentals of what would eventually change training in professional sports, specifically the National Football League – clean and jerks, bench press, and squats.

One of Ward's mentors on Muscle Beach was a guy named Vic Tanny, the man who developed and expanded America's first chain of workout facilities. Another guy who Ward worked out with at Muscle Beach was Don Wildman, who later went on to develop Bally's Total Fitness and became a multi-millionaire.

The original Muscle Beach was mysteriously bulldozed in 1959, and a number of theories exist as to why the city unceremoniously leveled its existence. One theory was a number of the bodybuilders were accused of raping underage girls there, so the city deemed the site a nuisance. The incident involved consensual sex between an adult and a minor, nonetheless statutory rape; charges in that case were dropped. The second and more widely accepted theory was that, by 1959 – long after Ward had graduated from Burbank High School and college, the area had begun to attract a "bad element" and the city wanted to clean it up to make way for parking in what was a rapidly growing area of Los Angeles.

Weight training would return to this area as much of the original Muscle Beach equipment resurfaced in a neighborhood basement called "The Dungeon." And, eventually, weight lifting in this region took off again in the '60s when the likes of bodybuilder Joe Gold made it popular. Gold would eventually start his own gym – Gold's Gym.

"Everybody I saw when I was there – Vic Tanny or all of those guys I saw working out on the beaches – those are the guys I duplicated," Ward recounts. "All of the stuff that those guys were talking about there – lifting, what to put in your body, vitamins – that's where I learned it."

A new "Muscle Beach Venice" was eventually erected two miles south of the original site where it has become a Mecca for bodybuilders.

The '60s and '70s are often called the Golden Era of bodybuilding. This era produced the likes of Arnold Schwarzenegger and a cult classic documentary called *Pumping Iron* – a film that chronicled the efforts of men pursuing the 1975 title of Mr. Olympia. All of it made lifting weights chic, popular, and cool; the film took it off the beaches, out of the basements, and into the mainstream all over the United States.

Right around this time, Bob Ward took the fundamental concepts he learned on the beach in Southern California into a weight room in Dallas, bringing these basics to professional football and eventually professional sports.

• • • •

Shortly after Ward graduated in January of 1951 from Burbank High School, he and a friend and football teammate, Chuck McCalmont, made a plan: They would join the Marines. That year, the U.S. had joined the fight against the Soviet-backed invasion of South Korea by the Democratic People's Republic of Korea in the north. Ward and McCalmont, like so many young men of their generation were both fueled and inspired by the hundreds of thousands of men who fought in World War II. They did not want to miss this opportunity to fight for their country. And a lot of their friends had been in the National Guard, even called up to active duty – despite the fact they were still in high school.

Both he and McCalmont were standing outside of the latter's house one afternoon laying out their plans to join the military and the war. McCalmont's father heard some of this chatter and came outside. Mr. McCalmont looked at the two teenage boys and said: "Wait a minute – go on into the house. I have a gun. Go get it, and you can shoot yourselves."

McCalmont was a veteran, and he knew that a teenaged boy's romanticized version of war was not how it played out in real life.

Ward admits, "As a stupid young kid who has no idea of what war is really like, you think you want to test yourself in that environment – yeah, I wanted to go. I had no idea what it was really like." Because he lived in an era where people, specifically returning soldiers from WWII, did not talk about "those things" that happened in the war, no one told him what war was actually like.

If he could help it, there was no way Mr. McCalmont would allow these boys to go fight. Because Ward was not quite 18, he couldn't enlist yet anyway, but he could go to college. The assistant football coach at Whitworth College (now Whitworth University) was dating the daughter of the minister at a local church, and he knew Ward and his buddy. The coach told them about Whitworth, which was how Bob Ward found his college of choice. Mr. McCalmont drove his son and Ward nearly 1,200 miles from Southern California to Spokane, Washington, to both attend Whitworth College and stay out of any war. Ironically, Ward completed college while McCalmont left after just one semester to join the Marines.

Ward would attend the then NAIA-school on an athletic scholarship that would cover nearly all of the costs; whatever he could not pay was made up for with a job on campus. One of his jobs was to pass out Bibles during chapel every week.

At Whitworth, Ward unknowingly laid the foundation for his career by simply never sitting still. He majored in physical education; became captain of the football team; earned NAIA All-American and all-conference honors as a fullback in football; threw the shot put, placing in the NAIA national meet in Abilene; and was a decathlete. He did summer jobs in an Alaskan sawmill, life guarded at a pool, and did some factory work. He also met his future wife, Joyce. To complete this Norman Rockwell painting, Joyce was a cheerleader. Ever the romantic, when Bob proposed to Joyce, he did it the old-fashioned way – over the phone.

The "C" student in high school who screwed around too much transformed himself into an A/B student during his college and university graduate years.

Bob's younger brother Paul, who would later go on to earn his PED from Indiana and become one of the most respected track coaches in the nation, wanted to go to college but didn't have the money. One afternoon, Paul was on the phone with his older brother when Bob asked him if he really wanted to go to college.

"Bob – *I don't have the money*," Paul answered.

Bob told his football coach – Jim Lounsberry – that his younger brother was the quarterback for the Burbank football team. That was about all it took for Lounsberry; he told Paul he could come to Whitworth with a scholarship.

After Paul Ward followed Bob to Whitworth, the youngest Ward brother, Maurice, eventually went there as well. All three earned their degrees from Whitworth.

Somewhere in college, Bob Ward quickly learned that people thought he was smart because of his constant need to expand his vocabulary. He liked the attention as well as the perception that he was intelligent because his vocabulary was large. One of the Whitworth football trainers even nicknamed him "Words Ward."

Ward's career at Whitworth was so distinguished he was inducted into the Whitworth's Heritage Gallery Hall of Fame in 1992.

• • • •

In the early spring of 1953, Ward received his official draft notice from the draft board.

Like any young man of that era, he was not going to deny his duty and desire to serve his country. He wanted to go to war, but the Korean War was *not* World War II. America was exhausted from the prolonged but victorious war against the Japanese and the Germans, which ended in 1945; the thirst for combat and a win against communism had not stirred the same type of patriotism and emotions as the previous war. The duration of this conflict was considerably shorter without the nation-wide support; fears of World War III between the U.S. and the North Koreans, indirectly the Soviets, and potentially even the Chinese prompted President Harry S. Truman to agree to a draw at the 38th Parallel on the peninsula that is Korea. Although the conflict ended in July 1953, the Cold War would only heighten, and indirectly impact Bob Ward and his pioneering studies and theories, for the next few decades.

Ward wanted to join a fight that had ended, in his estimation, prematurely. But there was nowhere to fight. He, nonetheless, joined the Marines and was placed in Platoon's Leader's Class. The Korean conflict ended shortly after he was technically drafted in 1953, but Ward would remain in the active service until 1957. He trained in Quantico, Virginia – where he also played for the Marines' base football team, ran for the track team, and would quickly learn to loathe the brutal humidity in Northern Virginia.

"I was a Candy Store Marine," he acknowledges. "I was in the Marines, and I served my country, which is something that is very important to me. I honor and I cherish it, but I never served on the front lines. I never got shot at. I was never in Korea or Vietnam. My timing was such I just missed it. The guys who went there – they are the ones who are the real heroes. They did the real work. They gave it all up."

Even when his time in the service was over, he remained in the Reserves until 1971, attaining the rank of Major with a Military Occupational Specialty (MOS) in artillery.

By the time Ward attained his degree from Whitworth in 1955, he had decided what he wanted to do – teach and coach. He also wanted to keep

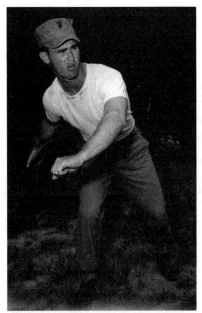

playing football before, or in conjunction with, his career as a teacher and a coach. Two years after his college career ended, he got his chance.

The New York Football Giants offered Ward a shot. Just before Ward was to report to the Marines in Quantico, Virginia, he received the word and was allowed to go to nearby Willamette University in Salem, Oregon; this was the site of the Giants' training camp where Ward would test himself against professional football players for a tryout. Some of the players in camp for the New York Giants included Frank Gifford, Kyle Rote, and Sam Huff. Also on that team was Dick Nolan, who would

U.S. Marine Platoon Leader's Class –
Bob Ward was a member of the United
States Marines in 1953.

later go on to become an NFL head coach and assistant with Ward on the Cowboys. The two most significant names on that Giants' team, however, were not players.

The defensive coordinator and defensive backs coach, who also served as the team's punter, was a quiet Texan named Tom Landry; three years after this training camp, Landry would accept the position of head coach of the Dallas Cowboys. Because Ward was a running back and Landry a defensive coach, the two men seldom, if ever, crossed paths. But, to Ward, what stood out about Tom Landry then was his quiet commanding presence.

The other notable name from this Giants team was nothing like Landry, other than he was a visionary and had a military background, as so many men of that generation did. This other notable name was not quiet in the least. He was an eruption of emotion. Unlike Landry, Ward saw this coach every day. The backfield coach who was also listed as the team's offensive coordinator was none other than Vince Lombardi. For roughly six weeks, Ward's position coach was the man the NFL would later name its championship trophy after – the iconic head coach of the Green Bay Packers, a man whose last name is synonymous with old-school football and winning.

"Coach Lombardi came out of West Point. He had this great, booming voice," Ward describes. "He was an un-equivocator. He was very competent and had this great delivery. He was a very persuasive individual – right or wrong, he got you to believe in his convictions. He was persuasive because of his confidence and knowing what he wanted to get done. He would yell at you, but he had this way that you wanted to do whatever he said because he was so convinced that his was the best way."

"But he never yelled at me," Ward chuckles. "…because I was perfect."

Of course, Ward was not perfect, but he was invited back after his Marine Corps duty was complete. Shortly thereafter, he reported to Quantico, Virginia for active duty. Bob tried out for the Giants again in 1957, but left during that camp because of a foot injury. That and the emotional draw of his wife and newborn daughter was difficult to ignore.

He had briefly talked to a scout once about trying out with the Dallas Cowboys in 1960, but that never came to fruition. Bob eventually made his way back to the state of Washington to start his post-playing career life, but he never was quite able to quit playing. In 1958, he had one more tryout with the

British Columbia Lions of the Canadian Football League; there he suffered a knee injury and was released.

"I was disappointed for a while because I wanted to play pro football and trained really hard to become a pro football player."

• • • •

By the time his football-playing career was over, Bob Ward had dodged all of the potential life-changing traps and potholes his formative years handed him. He was not into America's burgeoning drug scene, much of which was flowering in nearby Seattle when he was living in the area after college. Like so many of his generation, he did smoke cigarettes occasionally, though he quit in the '60s. Despite his time in the military, he had unintentionally avoided serving in Korea or Vietnam. He had not jumped into a bottle of whiskey or fallen in love with beer as a crutch – which was fortunate considering his family history. He had put himself through college. He had achieved considerable success despite the awful odds presented to him as a youth. He had met his wife, Joyce, with whom he would spend the rest of his life and have two daughters.

If he wasn't going to be able to play football, then at least he would be around those who could and help them improve in any capacity. He had figured out a way to take all of the experiences life had handed him and pass it down to others without crushing them.

He found his calling.

When Ward was coaching at Buena Park High School in 1965, there was a teenager throwing the shot put and discus at nearby Sunny Hills High School. Ward had seen Dave Murphy throw before, and he invited him to workout that summer with his guys. "I am this 15 or 16 year old kid, and I am looking at just this total stud; he was a guy that just looked great and could lift anything," Murphy remembered about first meeting Ward. "He could bench press 400 pounds. He could do back flips. He could do the pole vault. And, at that time, he was also going to Indiana to earn his doctorate. I was just so taken with his personality. He was such a role model."

As a high school senior, Murphy had athletic scholarship offers from nearly every major program in the country – UCLA, California, Ohio State, Michigan, Texas, USC. As a senior, his shot put distance of 67 feet, two inches set a new state record that would last until 1980. He could go anywhere he wanted to go save for one tiny problem. "My grades were terrible," he admitted.

Once those schools saw his terrible grades, the scholarship offers died. Unprompted and on his own time, Ward went to Murphy's home and knocked on the front door. His father answered, and Ward introduced himself. "What can I do to help?" Ward asked.

By the time Murphy graduated from high school, Ward had accepted the position as assistant track coach at nearby Fullerton Community College to work with a man who would go on to become one of the most distinguished track coaches in U.S. history – Tom Tellez. Murphy was not accepted into any four-year schools, so he followed Ward there.

"He made me pick myself up," Murphy said. "I did not realize until I worked with Bob that I was a weak competitor. I would easily crumble under pressure. He got me to be tough. I was down about myself and he knew it was necessary to grow up and to be a man and to get tough. He did not baby me at all."

After two good years at Fullerton, Murphy had the necessary grades; the scholarship offers that had once vanished returned. He accepted the offer from USC.

In 1970, Dave Murphy earned All-American NCAA Division I status in the discus and the shot put. He earned his degree in physical education and kinesiology.

"He was my role model," Murphy affirmed. "The guy I wanted to be was Bob Ward."

• • • •

Either consciously or subconsciously, Ward has deliberately tried to help those around him improve both the mind and the body for a simple reason: He was good at it. He was good at it because he saw it from conventional and unconventional sides. In a sense, Bob Ward had figured out how to help people without taking the time to sit down and figure it out. He had done it simply; he just kept moving. For the next several decades, he would spend his professional existence helping others figure out how to keep moving and improving, too.

CHAPTER 3

BILLION-DOLLAR
INDUSTRY

*"Competition is warfare. Mostly it is played by
prescribed rules – there is sort of a Geneva Convention
for competition – but it's thorough and often brutal."*
– Andrew S. Grove, former President & CEO of Intel Corp.

Jimmy Johnson did not care to understand what Bob Ward was doing, and in truth, all of the information Ward had compiled to show the head coach of the Dallas Cowboys only served to emphasize what was already obvious: In 1989, the New York Giants were a better football team than the Dallas Cowboys. Nothing Ward could do or could have done was going to change that. Bob is not a palindrome for God.

It was not as if Jimmy Johnson didn't know what he was doing or that he was a dumb coach incapable of listening. History shows he was everything but. He won a pair of Super Bowl championships with the Dallas Cowboys and built a team that would win three total in the '90s, thus securing his legacy as a man whose methods were easily validated as effective.

During their argument in 1990, Jimmy didn't want spreadsheets or any "damn analysis" from his weight lifting coach. He wanted damn big. He wanted damn fast. He didn't care if his first strength and conditioning coach was considered a visionary. The irony is some of Jimmy's ideas and concepts about football were as revolutionary as Ward's were about strength training and performance enhancement. Jimmy was one of the first NFL coaches to embrace and emphasize speed everywhere among his defensive players; he implemented the frequent rotation of fresh defensive players into the game. Ward believed in analyzing data to maximize performance and trying a variety of new methods to go beyond what the physical ceiling was considered to be.

What Jimmy was able to do on the field with his players, Ward was able to do with analytics and workouts.

Dr. Bob Ward believed in *Moneyball* before *Moneyball* was a thing, a slogan, or a verb in sports vernacular. *Moneyball*, the best-selling book by writer Michael Lewis published in 2003, is permanently attached to baseball and specifically the Oakland Athletics and general manager Billy Beane. In 2011, actor Brad Pitt played Beane in the Hollywood film production of the book that made the concepts *Moneyball* introduced even bigger. *Moneyball* is often associated with evaluating players based almost exclusively on statistical evidence and extensive situational analysis, which is something Bob Ward had done with the Dallas Cowboys more than 25 years earlier.

The *Moneyball* of the Oakland A's was a bold solution to a complicated problem, or as Ward would say, how Billy Beane found a way to cut his team's Gordian Knot.

Why *Moneyball* generated such a wide appeal outside of just baseball fans and seamheads is because, at its root, it's all about finding and creating value – in fact, these ideas were and are often used in college-level economics courses for that very reason. It is all about looking at something in a different manner that bucks conventional methods. It is about specific situations and quantified, probability outcome.

When it comes to sports in general, *Moneyball* may as well be synonymous with going against traditional thought by committing to a complete immersion in data and statistical research. As Ward believes, "The answers are always in the numbers. The key is *finding* the numbers," he explains. "Then, you just have to figure out what the numbers mean."

While it is not as simple as a math equation, there now exist methods and scores of data and research to create better results. The data is indisputable that, in some cases, *Moneyball* principles do work and are a dramatic improvement over previous methods.

Dr. Bob Ward was *"Moneyball*-ing" strength and conditioning before anybody else in the NFL; he was one of the first to do so in American athletics overall. Using the Dallas Cowboys as his laboratory and the players as his lab rats, he would test, research, and scrutinize player performance both in the gym and on the field looking for ways to improve performance, looking for answers to the performance equation. The amount of statistical data he kept is staggering and virtually unheard for a man in his position in the '70s.

Today, they're all doing it. Today, everyone in competitive and professional sports is trying to *Moneyball* their way to winning.

• • • •

If your favorite sports team doesn't have a "Bob Ward" on its payroll, that organization either doesn't care about winning or is horrendously cheap. When Ward began coaching the Dallas Cowboys in 1976, the position of conditioning coach had existed but was not a full-time job with benefits. He was the first full-time NFL conditioning coach to be treated like a regular coach with full-time benefits and a pension. His presence with the Cowboys would inspire nearly every other professional sports team to add someone just like him. When Ward left his job as Fullerton Community College track coach for the Cowboys, it was at a time when strength training as well as muscle building and conditioning were still in their infancy in professional sports.

When Bob Ward was playing youth football in the '40s, he had been told *not* to lift weights. By the '50s and certainly the '60s, that mindset had begun to change. In fact, some football players as early as the '60s may have been experimenting with anabolic steroids. But, outside of a few sports, namely football and Olympic sports that catered to larger men, weight lifting was something athletes simply didn't do. Along those same lines, nutrition and hydration were on the radar of almost no one at that time.

Former Texas Rangers outfielder Tom Grieve, who played nine MLB seasons from 1970 to 1979 and would later serve as the team's general manager, effectively encapsulated what strength and conditioning was like in that era in professional sports in every sport but football:

"There was no weight room when I was with the Texas Rangers. At all. It did not exist. They told you *not* to lift weights. We didn't put a weight room in here until 1981 or 1982. I played basketball in the offseason, and I might have jogged. Maybe you ran. That was it. That was 10 to 15, 40 or 50-yard wind sprints. No one ran for aerobic results. I might go for a run on the street for a mile, and I felt like I was running a marathon. I was thinking, 'I know I am working harder than anybody else.'

"We would get to spring training, and when guys took the baseball out of the bag it was the first time they had picked up a ball since the previous season ended. You could just see how sore guys were.

"The whole thought was – don't do anything to impede normal baseball movement. That's why we didn't lift weights. No one thought to do it because that was the way it was always done. The fear was that if you lifted weights, you would be muscle bound. It was presented to us from old baseball people that didn't know what they were talking about. Eventually, it did become a science because of men like Bob Ward, Tom House and a lot of other guys."

Tom House was the former Texas Rangers pitching coach who once had his pitchers, including Nolan Ryan, practice by throwing footballs. House's name and reputation would eventually grow and expand to the point where he became synonymous with throwing mechanics. His clientele would eventually include some guy who's had moderate success at football – Tom Brady.

"Why wouldn't you want a stronger body?" Grieve asked. "It was stupid what we were doing. You are going to be stronger, and your baseball movements will be stronger and quicker. I remember I was with the Mets in 1978 and [manager] Joe Torre hired a guy, who was on me all the time about lifting weights. I am thinking, 'I am *not* doing this.' Finally one day I agreed to do it. He had me doing things they wouldn't dream of doing today – dead lifts, presses, stuff like that. Afterwards, I was dead. I couldn't even move. I never went back in.

"As far as eating, the six years I was with the Rangers the only food that was in the clubhouse was a keg of beer, and a big thing of pretzels and potato chips. In 1974, they added a microwave so you could have a hot dog. That was like having a gourmet meal. Now, they practically have restaurants in every clubhouse. You can have an organic meal any time you want here. The teams have chefs that prepare the food.

"It really never did make sense to me that being stronger would not help you as a baseball player. I just always had accepted what they said and what they told me. But it did seem to be that baseball needed to take a step forward and out of the dark ages. It was time for it."

Catcher Mike Scioscia began a 13-year major league career with the Los Angeles Dodgers, right around the same time Grieve's career was ending. Scioscia broke in with the Dodgers in 1980, which is just about the time baseball began to look more closely at the area that would eventually transform the sport in America – the weight room.

"Nobody lifted weights," said Scioscia, who has had a long tenure as the manager of the Los Angeles Angels during a time when he saw weight lifting – and the rampant use of steroids and performance enhancing drugs – alter the game and its record books.

"Remember when Nautilus machines came out? They came about the time [when Scioscia reached the Major Leagues]. They were supposed to be revolutionary.

"Baseball had always been considered a non-lifting sport for various reasons. I know it would have helped me because I historically had very good first halves (of a season), and then in the second half wasn't that good. That was even in the minor leagues. With the advances of strength and conditioning, we understand that baseball is a sport that does need stamina."

By the mid-'80s, strength training and muscle mass had begun to rapidly expand throughout nearly every sport. The weight room was no longer just for weight lifters and body builders.

Veteran NBA head coach Rick Carlisle, who has coached the Detroit Pistons, Indiana Pacers and won an NBA title with the Dallas Mavericks in 2011, played at the University of Virginia in the '80s. He had a three-year career with the Boston Celtics from 1984 to 1987, and he played two more years with the New York Knicks and New Jersey Nets before he entered coaching.

"We were lifting some weights. My strength and conditioning program was not a lot different than they are today," Carlisle said. "Some of the techniques and approaches have changed as research has gotten more sophisticated. There has been a lot of study on flexibility, and the type of strength that is important. And recovery.

"Today, what you have is a lot more stuff on core training and balance work. We did not have that in the '80s. That balance work came from you balancing dumbbells. It was a lot different. If you were using Nautilus stuff, it was different, too; now things are much more geared towards balance and core. There is more stretch band work, which makes the negative part of the exercise the more critical part. A lot of things have changed, but the need for strength and conditioning has not. What has changed is the research and what we know about it."

The Dallas Cowboys specifically brought on Ward as a "Strength and Conditioning Coach." That was the title, but when he was hired, he was handed carte blanche by head coach Tom Landry. The Cowboys allowed Ward to do *whatever* he felt necessary. The Cowboys hired him because he was good in a field that was growing at a time when the organization was ahead on everything.

Previously, everyone in similar jobs had been "muscle guys" whose mission it was to get guys big, jacked. While the knowledge and science around physical performance had increased tenfold since the advent of the first Super Bowl in 1967, the application of those advances had not been universally applied to the NFL.

For the better part of the '60s and the '70s, pro sports remained rooted in quaint and modest upbringings that started mostly in the '50s, long before technology began to become a societal constant and the financial incentive had not crossed into the millions of dollars. The cable TV revolution would not happen until the '80s, meaning ESPN and its global cultural impact on sports was years away. The NBA was still on tape delay. MLB was easily the most popular professional sport in the U.S. while hockey and soccer were niche sports. Boxing and horseracing still enjoyed a large piece of the American sports market. But the NFL and college football were the growing monsters.

When Ward started with the Cowboys, it was a time when the participants themselves did not train year round. It was not totally uncommon for football players to have a second job in the offseason. Back then, sports were not necessarily a "career path" as much as they were a fun diversion until you decided to do something else with your life.

What sports looked like in the mid-'70s hardly resembled the global, billion-dollar titan it is three decades later:

In 1975...

— the NHL and NBA had 18 teams, respectively.

— MLB had 24 teams.

— the NFL had 26 teams.

— there was no Major League Soccer.

— there was no professional sports league for women.

In 2015...

— the NHL and NBA both feature 30 franchises.

— MLB has 30 teams.

— the NFL has 32 teams.

— there are 20 Major League Soccer franchises.

— the Women's National Basketball Association has 12 teams, and the league has existed since 1996.

Since Ward interviewed with the Dallas Cowboys in 1976, the number of professional minor league sports has exploded, and now dozens and dozens of countries spend millions of dollars to train Olympic athletes.

There are a number of factors that led to this global sports expansion, top among them the advent and proliferation of cable television, the need for live programming, and the growth of discretionary entertainment spending. When Ward entered the NFL, competition was casually fierce; nothing like the savage, cutthroat mentality of 21st century sports. The origins of that modern struggle begin in player training, evaluation, and preparation all with the intent to improve however possible, no matter how fractional the gains.

By the time Ward left the Cowboys in 1990, pro sports – specifically the NFL – was in the midst of a growth spurt that really hasn't stopped since. In 2015, the revenue of professional sports surpasses the economy of many nations.

If the position held by Dr. Bob Ward was an anomaly when he started with the Cowboys, it is common today.

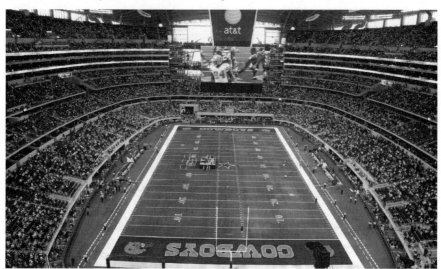

Interior view of the AT&T Stadium – formerly Cowboys Stadium – which was completed in May 2009. Maximum capacity with standing room is 105,000, a big jump from the 65,675 capacity of the Cowboys' former home, Texas Stadium.

- When the Dallas Mavericks played its first NBA season in 1980 – 81, the team listed five people who had to do with on-court performance, including one head coach and one assistant coach. For the 2014-15 season, the Dallas Mavericks employed 33 people who deal with on-court performance. They have a free throw shooting coach. Like most teams, they also employ a sports psychologist and a nutritionist.
- By comparison, in 2015, a few miles up the road from the Mavs in Dallas at Southern Methodist University – the Mustangs men's basketball team features a "support staff" just for that program with 15 positions. The women's basketball team has 11 positions.
- In 1975, under head coach Chuck Knox, the Los Angeles Rams featured two trainers on their staff and no strength coaches. They also had two scouts. By 2015, the Rams had moved to St. Louis and have 11 people who have the title of "scout." They also have three strength coaches and four trainers.
- The Ohio State Buckeyes, in their 2015 football program, list 19 coaches, four of whom are listed as "assistant strength & conditioning coach." The Buckeyes also have an assistant athletic director for "Football Sports Performance."

The year Ward officially joined the Cowboys, head coach Tom Landry had a staff featuring eight assistants as well as two trainers and an equipment manager. The team also had seven scouts, which was among the most in the NFL at the time.

For the 2014 season, the Cowboys listed 17 positions associated with personnel, which is basically scouting – they even staff a full-time position titled "Combine Scout" and have 16 assistant coaches.

Today, there are now so many "Bob Ward" types in sports, he would simply blend in with the rest.

Consider this coaching roster for starters: When the Philadelphia Eagles hired Chip Kelly away from the University of Oregon in January of 2013, he too hired a man named Shaun Huls, who had been the strength and conditioning coach – and combatives coordinator – for Navy Special Warfare. Kelly and the Eagles gave Huls the title of "Sports Science Coordinator." They eventually renamed his title "Director of Sports Science Coordinator and Re-Conditioning." In the spring of 2015, the Eagles hired a man named James Hanisch as "High Performance Analyst"; Hanisch had a similar job in the Australian Football League. They also hired J.P. Crowley Hanlon as "Logistics Coordinator."

Sports has become such a massive business with so much potential money to be made that innumerable people want to be a "Dr. Bob Ward" because teams routinely hire one in the name of finding any edge over the competition. Since the Cowboys paved the way by hiring Dr. Bob Ward, nearly every team in virtually every sport has looked for their own version of him.

Ward's Words
The Secret to Getting into Shape

As a former NFL conditioning coach, I am often asked, "How do I lose weight?" Or "What should I do to get into shape?" The truth is, there is no one secret ingredient to doing either one.

It's simple – Be smart with how you eat, exercise, and don't over-do anything. You likely already know what to do – eating cheeseburgers, French fries, and drinking beer are not going to make the impact you want. Even if you exercise routinely, you can't out-exercise your mouth.

There are three other things I've learned about people who get into shape and live a healthy lifestyle:

1. *They are passionate about it, so they want to do it without any added incentive.*
2. *They are scared into doing it; for instance, a doctor tells a person they will die if they don't lose weight, eat better, and "get into shape." Their incentive is clear, so they do it.*
3. *They teach themselves how to do it.*

This does not mean if you are not passionate about it or haven't had a doctor scare you to death, that you can't lose weight or get into shape. You can, but you must have a plan. You will not go anywhere if you just go to the gym and "workout for an hour." Before you go to the gym, know what it is you want to achieve, have a goal. You must have a goal if you work out. If it's simply to lose weight, have a plan. If it's to get bigger biceps, figure out how to do it; don't just do a bunch of bicep curls. If it's to run a marathon, find the right training program.

Whatever your goal, do not be afraid to lift weights as a part of your workout; the fear that lifting weights will make you bigger and bulky is not true. Lifting weights at high repetition will increase your metabolism and burn calories better than 30 minutes on the treadmill at the same speed.

Be patient. These types of changes take many days and months before you will see the desired results and be able to permanently change the pattern of behavior so it becomes a more permanent habit. The more you do it, the more you exercise, the better prepared you will be to do more exercise. It is crucial that before you begin you address the following:

1. **Purpose.** *Have a good goal that is not easily achieved, but is realistic. Give yourself goals that you can attain, so you can taste success. Success leads to more success.*

2. **Principle.** *Develop guides or plans to achieve the goal.*

3. **Integrity.** *Be true to your plans. Take the actions necessary to achieve the goals.*

4. **Independence.** *The ability to be free because you paid the price of doing each step.*

What I am providing is the same thing I gave the Dallas Cowboys in 1976, and they followed it for several years with modifications. You are likely not a professional athlete, meaning you do not have three hours a day to workout like an NFL player does. But, if you take the principles of what is provided and modify them to your body and your needs, you can do it in less than one hour. You must first do a little bit of research – find a plan that works for you and your desires – and you must write it down. All of the research and experts agree with the point that you are much more likely to pursue something when you write it down. And when you do that, then you must follow it, and you can do it.

Once you set that, you can modify the following of what I implemented with the Dallas Cowboys:

1. **Warm-up**
   Nothing too strenuous, but something to break a sweat and simply get your blood flowing, increase your body temperature, and increase elasticity. Perhaps an easy run or jump rope for a few minutes.

2. **Flexibility exercises**
   This is all about increasing the range of movement and continuing to warm up the body. Examples include Achilles/calf/hip/shoulder neck circles; toe touches; roll (back-sides) feet overhead; roll-tucked position.

3. **Technique Drills, Spring & Jumping Drills**
   High knee, arm action; 40-75 yards

4. ***Main Workout***

   This is the portion where you get specific. This is where you train for the marathon, play football, play basketball, or whatever it is that you choose to pursue.

5. ***Warm-down***

   Nothing complicated. Easy jogging or just walking.

   I'm in my 80s, and I exercise three to five days a week at the gym. I have the advantage of having been passionate about exercising, movement, working out, and lifting weights since I was a kid. It gave me confidence and made me feel better about myself. It was never work for me to work out, or to lift weights. I loved doing it. I have been blessed by God to have these genes. I am flattered to hear I look much younger than I am, but that is because of these genes and that I take care of my body.

   You don't have to be scared to death or love exercising to be the ideal version of you. There is no such thing as, "It's too late." Have a purpose. Have a plan. Have a goal. Listen to your body. Start feeling better.

CHAPTER 4

THE LONG SHOT LANDS ON AMERICA'S TEAM

"We often miss opportunity because it's
dressed in overalls and looks like work."
– Thomas A. Edison

When Tom Landry called Bob Ward's house, the voice on the other end was not the man he wanted. The voice on the other end was not a man at all.

"Hello?" the high-pitched voice asked. "Bob Ward's Cookie Factory – which crumb would you like to speak to?"

This was not Bob Ward, nor was it his wife, Joyce. This was their youngest daughter, Erin.

"Who is it?" Erin's older sister, Shannon, asked.

Clearly unimpressed with the caller, Erin switched the phone from one shoulder to the other and shrugged, "Some guy named Tom Landry."

A football fan, Shannon stood up and quietly screamed – *"That's Tom Landry?'"*

Shannon grabbed the phone and immediately took the message. This was the phone call Bob Ward had been hoping for.

• • • •

Bob Ward was not the first choice to be the first full-time conditioning coach of the Dallas Cowboys. The first choice for this newly created position was a former colleague of Ward's, Tom Tellez. Tellez was a long-time track coach in Southern California, and in some circles, he is regarded as the finest track coach of any era.

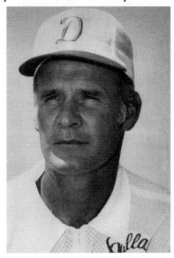

Dallas Cowboys head coach Tom Landry in 1976 – the year he hired Bob Ward.

In 1980, Tellez was named as one of the U.S. Olympic team track coaches, but was denied its fulfillment because the U.S. boycotted the 1980 Games in Moscow, a protest led by then President Jimmy Carter over the Soviet invasion of Afghanistan.

Like Ward, he was a part of the analytic movement in human performance that involved physiology and biomechanics.

Tellez had been offered the job by then-Cowboys vice president of personnel Gil Brandt and head coach Tom Landry.

"How they knew about me was because of Dick Vermeil," Tellez said, who worked with the future NFL Super Bowl-winning head coach when Vermeil was the head coach at UCLA. "Dick was the ultimate at not leaving any stone unturned."

Tellez and Vermeil were chatting one day in the UCLA athletic offices when the football coach shocked the track coach: "I want you to talk to my team," Vermeil told Tellez.

"Are you sure?" Tellez replied, almost confused. This was not the norm for a football coach. "I may say a lot of things that are different than what you say or your assistants say."

"Talk to them. I want you to talk to the players and the coaches," he repeated.

Vermeil was renowned for trying anything to motivate players and finding any technique or method to give his team the edge. He was also a renowned workaholic.

"Dick had a staff that was loaded with good teachers, and their minds were open to different ideas," Tellez said. "And they liked what I was doing with 'maximum performance.' At the time, I was really more into running and what Bob was doing was more strength-based research. But we were both looking for maximum performance."

Maximum Performance involved five basics:

1. Strength training
2. Endurance training
3. Speed training
4. Flexibility
5. Mental concentration

*According to Tellez, there is also a sixth, "Rest. That is probably the most important."

It would be nearly impossible today to find a training program on the professional level that does not include these six basics.

"I talked to the UCLA team about how they all fit into a program and what they should do to get ready on a weekly basis; it's not like track where they have a build up to the NCAA championships or just a meet at the end of the season," Tellez explained. "In football, every week is important. Every week is the Olympics. You are not building up to a final game. You have an Olympics every week, and the training tactics have to be built-in before the season starts and throughout the season to prepare for each game."

That part of the job with a football team, and potentially with the Dallas Cowboys, appealed to Tellez. The part that did not appeal to him was the prospect of leaving the college environment to work with pro athletes. Some coaches are "college guys" and some are "pro guys." The egos are different, as is the pain-in-the-ass meter. Tellez was a "college guy," no doubt.

About the decision he made, "I interviewed with the Cowboys, and it was intriguing, but I knew I wanted to be a track coach. That's what I wanted to do. I had been offered the head coaching position at Houston, and I just felt that I would be a better fit. I liked the college environment too much. I didn't think I would work that well with the pros."

Ward had asked Tellez if he would mind giving Coach Tom Landry his name, but he never said anything more than, "Have him call me!"

When Tellez called the Dallas Cowboys to inform them he was going to accept the position at Houston, he did offer one suggestion. "The guy you really should call and interview is Bob Ward," Tellez told Tom Landry. "He would be good."

Ward had known Tellez for years and almost followed his career path step for step in Southern California. He followed Tellez as a coach at Buena Park High School in the early '60s and took over as head track coach and assistant football coach. Tellez hired Ward to be his assistant at Fullerton Community College in 1965, and when he became the head coach at UCLA in 1969, Ward took over his spot. They were both former small college football players turned track coaches who did extensive research on athletic performance enhancement.

"I knew Bob would be a better fit for that job than I would," Tellez said. "I had approached maximum performance from a running standpoint, and Bob had approached it from the strength training standpoint. The hard part was that Bob didn't have a name. I did not know if they would give him the job because he was not at a big university. But, in terms of his personality and his work and his studies, he was an ideal fit for where football was going. He had written papers, he had his doctorate, and he had done research, but he was at Fullerton Community College."

Tellez made the right call for his career. He was at Houston for 22 years and coached U.S. Olympic medalists Carl Lewis, Leroy Burrell, and Joe DeLoach among scores of other successful sprinters.

• • • •

As the coach of a junior college program, despite his academic and athletic credentials, Ward was a long shot. The fact that the California Junior College system was loaded with highly skilled athletes and was well regarded academically didn't matter much since Fullerton was not a big name four-year program, like UCLA, Ohio State, or Texas.

Ward had met Tom Landry before, but he was not sure if the head coach of the Dallas Cowboys would have remembered that meeting. In 1955 before joining the USMC and later after he left the USMC in 1957, Ward had a tryout with the New York Giants when Landry was an assistant coach. Ward was never sure if Landry remembered him from his brief tryouts with the Giants, but he assumed the answer was no.

When the Cowboys did call, they didn't immediately offer the job. Ward had to fly out from Los Angeles to Dallas to go through a two-day interview process with Landry, team president Tex Schramm, and the assistant coaches as well as meet with a psychologist, Dr. Ray Fletcher. Ward stayed at Holiday Inn near the Cowboys' headquarters, which at the time were located just north of downtown Dallas and close to SMU.

He immediately liked Landry and Schramm.

In jobs such as these, it is doubtful the Cowboys looked too closely at his resume even if he had two specific credentials that separated him from just about any other candidate at that time. Few men in his position back then would have had a graduate degree, and virtually none of them would have had a doctorate. Dr. Bob Ward had both, not to mention a knack for innovation.

• • • •

As a former decathlete, Ward was well-versed in all of the skills required in track and field. Given his strong build, he tended to be a bit better in the throwing events. In the '60s, when he was coaching at Fullerton, he began to fool around with techniques to throw the shot put. There simply had to be better way, and as it turns out, there was.

For decades, high jumpers all followed the same techniques in order to cross the bar – a straddle technique or a roll was deemed the best way. In the mid-'60s, American high jumper Richard Fosbury started to tinker with a different method to clear the bar. His coaches implored him not to try the head-first, back-to-the-bar method because it looked to be too dangerous. In 1968 at the Summer Olympics in Mexico City, Fosbury set the world record by clearing a height of 7 feet 4 ¼ inches to set a new Olympic record and win an Olympic gold medal. His new "dangerous" method is now known as "The Fosbury Flop," and it has since been emulated by anybody who wants to be a successful high jumper.

Around that time, Ward began to mess around with a different way to throw a discus or shot put. The more he did it and the more he studied it, he thought that if the thrower began to spin himself, it would create more momentum and energy to throw the shot, or disc, further.

Today, Ward is one of four men to be cited in this revolution: Toni Nett of Germany, Victor Alexeyev of the Soviet Union, Klement Kerssen Brock of Czechoslovakia, and Dr. Bob Ward are credited as the geniuses behind the "spin move" in the shot based on commonly used discus biomechanics.

"This was a case really of using analytics," Ward says, "all you had to do was just look at it – it made a lot more sense to generate momentum before you throw the shot or the discus. I would experiment with spinning when I was at Fullerton, and the more I did it, the farther I threw. You could see the actual improvements right there."

• • • •

Tellez made sure to mention this specific creation of Ward's to the Cowboys. What the Cowboys knew, thanks to Tellez, was enough to convince them to look at Bob Ward, but there were concerns and fears that had be addressed.

"I spent all morning taking these tests and talking to this psychologist. I took the Wonderlic test, too," Ward remembers. "The big thing they wanted to know about was how I dealt with African Americans. They really questioned me to try to find out if I was prejudiced."

Ward's mother and father both grew up in an era where racial prejudices were not uncommon, and Ward's generation certainly had experienced its share of unrest rooted in antiquated but still government-protected biases. "We had black athletes on the track teams that I coached and it wasn't like I had never been around blacks or minorities - like the 'Zoot Suits' in California in the '40s," he describes. "I didn't have any problem with it, but that was a big part of the interview."

The hardest part of the interview process to conceive was that Ward was not salivating at this job opportunity as the clichéd job of a lifetime. Today, there would be a line 50 miles long of qualified candidates eager to take this position. When the Cowboys offered the job in the spring of 1976, Ward was eager for a different job opportunity, but cautious about leaving Fullerton.

When the Dallas Cowboys offered Bob Ward the opportunity to become a full-time member of their staff, he didn't say no, but it wasn't a straight yes either. Ward's wife, Joyce, wanted to go. The idea did sound slightly enthralling to him, too, but Bob was more cautious. He had it too good teaching and coaching at Fullerton.

"I really did not want to give up my benefits," Ward explains. "I had tenure and good benefits at the school. And I had no real idea of what it was going to be like. I thought it would be a fickle thing to do. To me, I was using it as a test and an experiment. I knew how fragile the whole thing was." But, at the same time, he had been at Fullerton for a while, so he was up for a new challenge.

In today's world, it's hard to fathom a professional leaning toward remaining at his job at a junior college over the National Football League. Back then, the difference wasn't as staggering as one might think. Ward was being paid $17,000 at the time in a tenure-track job with benefits; in 2016, he would be making about $71,000. Leaving for the Dallas Cowboys then was not the financial boon that it is today. They offered him an annual starting salary of $21,000; that would be $88,847 in 2016. A decent raise, yes, but not like winning the lottery.

For Joyce, who was a dance teacher at Cypress College in the same Fullerton Community College District, this was not a difficult decision. The decision was to go. Right then. "It was not hard to move me. It was exciting," she recalls. "While he kept saying, 'I don't know – I want to see what it's like,' he did say, 'I gotta do this.' For Bob, he was always looking to expand – five years at anything was about it."

At the time, they had one daughter in college at their alma mater, Whitworth College, and another in middle school. The couple had previously been to Texas one time – Dallas in the early '70s. That was the extent of their knowledge of the state. Ward outlined an agreement that he would take the position on a trial-basis only. It would be for two years, and then he would re-evaluate his professional life. Fullerton agreed that he could take a two-year leave of absence without threatening his tenure or benefits.

When the Cowboys offered Ward the title of "Strength and Conditioning Coach," they were already well established as the leader in innovation in sports, both on and off the field. He was certainly familiar with the team; in 1960, the first year the franchise existed in the NFL, Ward interviewed with a scout about a potential tryout in California when he was teaching. So, Ward was familiar with the Cowboys, but he was not so well-versed in the extent of the franchise's innovation when it came to football and the business of football.

The Cowboys' had the first organized professional cheerleading squad; it's a unit that is now synonymous with professional sports cheerleading, complete with its own reality television show. The second home to the Dallas Cowboys – Texas Stadium – revolutionized the professional sports seating and in-game experience. The Cowboys were the first to offer suites, which could be custom furnished, and the first offer what are now called "Personal Seat Licenses" to patrons interested in season tickets. When it came to scouting, the Cowboys were the first keep an extensive log, cataloging every potential incoming prospect.

When it came to Ward's field of expertise, the Cowboys were first there, too.

• • • •

Before Ward arrived, if there was a painful way to lose a game, the Cowboys had perfected that as well.
- In 1966, the Cowboys lost the NFL Championship game against Green Bay by seven points in Dallas.
- In 1967, the Cowboys again lost the NFL Championship game, this time at Green Bay in the infamous "Ice Bowl" at Lambeau Field with a wind chill of minus 48 degrees. They lost in the final seconds of that game. In the fourth quarter, Dan Reeves, who would later become

a Cowboys assistant coach and NFL head coach, threw a 50-yard touchdown pass to give the Cowboys a 17-14 lead before they ultimately lost to the Packers, final score 21-17.

- In 1970, the Cowboys lost Super Bowl V by three points to the Baltimore Colts. In that game, the Cowboys had a 13-6 lead in the fourth only to blow it. The Colts scored the game-winning field goal with five seconds remaining in the game. This is the only Super Bowl in history where the game's Most Valuable Player came from the *losing* team – Cowboys linebacker Chuck Howley.

"We were always 'Next Year's Champion,'" said former Cowboys player and long-time assistant coach Dan Reeves. To become "This Year's Champion," something obviously needed to change.

Thanks to a then mostly unregulated NFL financial landscape and the money owner Clint Murchison – who did not skimp on anything – supplied, the Cowboys were the first to incentivize players to just work out at the team's facility.

"Coach Landry had the Cowboys pay us $50 a workout in the offseason if we did it there at the team's facility," Reeves said. "We were one of the first teams that started to do that – we had players stay with the team in the offseason. That was a tremendous advantage.

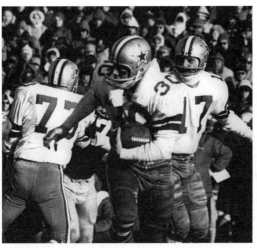

"That time we spent there working out together it built camaraderie and it carried over. It was just enough money for a guy to stay in Dallas in the offseason. And by doing that program, it did make us faster and stronger."

Photo Courtesy of Malcolm Emmons/USA TODAY

Dallas Cowboys running back Dan Reeves runs the ball against the Green Bay Packers during the 1967 NFL Championship game in Green Bay, Wisconsin. Dubbed the "Ice Bowl" and the coldest game in NFL history, the temperature was recorded at 13 below zero with a wind chill of minus 48 degrees.

According to Reeves, the team would test the players, which included the standing broad jump. If a guy could cover 10 feet, "He was considered a hell of an athlete," Reeves said. In 1973, the Cowboys had two guys who could do that – wide receiver Bob Hayes, a former Olympian whose presence in the NFL changed the entire league, and cornerback Mel Renfro. Both of these men were inducted into the Pro Football Hall of Fame; they were superior athletes who could broad jump over a barn without the training.

"When guys started to train in the offseason, you could see a difference when we tested. Before, in the case of the broad jump, the only guys that could do it were Mel and Bob. After we trained together, there were 12 to 15 guys that could do it. You could really see the offseason training together worked."

Not coincidentally, that was the first year the team had hired strength coach Alvin Roy away from the Kansas City Chiefs. Roy, considered by some to be the first professional strength coach to be hired by an NFL team, served under General George S. Patton in World War II and began his career with the American Football League's San Diego Chargers in 1963. The Chargers won the AFL championship in Roy's first season and reached the title game in each of the following seasons.

In 1968, Roy left San Diego to join the Kansas City Chiefs. The next year, the Chiefs won the Super Bowl.

In 1973, Roy left Kansas City to join the Dallas Cowboys. That season, the "Next Year's Champion" became "This Year's Champion" when the Cowboys won their first Super Bowl.

After the 1975 season, Kansas City Chiefs head coach Hank Stramm called Roy and offered him a $14,000 raise. The Cowboys declined to match it. Before leaving, Alvin Roy wrote a note and sent it to Gil Brandt. It simply said, "I sold my soul for a $14,000 raise."

"We didn't fire him or dismiss him. He just left for a raise," Brandt said. "That's when we went looking for somebody else."

When Roy left, the Cowboys had clearly seen enough to know a man in his position made a difference, but they wanted something else, something better.

• • • •

Asking Tom Tellez to join the Dallas Cowboys was typical of what the franchise did at that time under Schramm's direction. They were either the first or right behind those who were first. Tellez was a logical choice. Schramm was the biggest believer that winning sold everything, a belief more easily achieved with a big spending owner. Schramm was known to say when it came to marketing, spend that money on scouting, on finding talent.

The Cowboys' success in this era of the '70s is the single biggest reason the franchise remains one of the most popular and profitable in the world.

"He never took any money out of the team," said Brandt. "In fairness to a lot of other teams, we were able to do things because we had the money. And Tex loved to spend money."

Because of the money not taken out by owner Clint Murchison, the team continually re-invested in itself. The way the Dallas Cowboys viewed football was not like a sport. "We viewed it like a business," Brandt said. "We treated it like a business before anybody else did. We wanted to find a way to do it quicker, better, and less expensive."

The Cowboys were the first to sponsor, or suggest, Pro Days at college campuses, which are now routine at nearly every college football program in the nation. The team would wine and dine college head and assistant coaches all over the country, all in the name of obtaining information on players. They would give pins, or just stuff, to college equipment guys because it might have paid off with a piece of information on a player or two.

This was long before the days of more restrictive player signing practices. The Cowboys would bring in scores of undrafted players and pay to house them at apartments, keeping them in town year-round. Or they would give a player an advance of $5,000, provided it was put down on a house in the Dallas area. "It allowed us to keep rookies close and to work them out all the time. Some of those guys still live in those houses we helped put the $5,000 down towards" Brandt said. "We knew the only way we would get better was to be creative, and that was a way to do it."

The other way was to embrace technology and computers. When Schramm worked with CBS in the early '60s, he saw first-hand the potential of computers and technology. He had seen that IBM had put a computer chip into a steer, which allowed the tracking of the bull's movements. The Cowboys would eventually visit Delta, UPS, etc., to learn about similar logistical technology.

"UPS would try to come up with routes for its drivers that would be right-turns only," Brandt said. "They had it down to where they figured out how many hours their drivers wasted on left turns."

Player evaluation back then could be maddeningly inefficient. For instance, the Cowboys once drafted a cornerback based on the hunch of a defensive coach who had seen him work out at a small school in Kentucky. He looked great, and in practice, he was fine. But, when the game started, the guy was lost. "Why did we draft this guy?" coach Tom Landry asked. "Did you watch the game film on him?"

The Cowboys' assistant coach admitted that he had not seen any tape on the player. That was the last time the assistant coaches were permitted to have any influence on the Draft for the Cowboys. What the team wanted to do was to evaluate strictly on performance, rather than on emotion. What the Cowboys needed, and what eventually every other team would emulate, was a system of collecting data and grading players.

"Every housewife could tell you who the top 10 percent and the bottom 10 percent of the players were coming out of college," Brandt said. "The trick was finding that 80 percent."

In 1962, Schramm reached out to IBM about developing a system to collect, store, and evaluate player data. It eventually led him to a subsidiary of IBM and a man named A. Salam Qureishi – a computer programmer from Uttar Pradesh in Northern India. The man did not know American football and spoke with a heavy accent, but he knew computers and he knew baseball.

"I had learned to enjoy baseball because of its similarity to cricket," Qureishi once told *Sports Illustrated*. "Now, I think American football is easily the most scientific game ever invented."

Qureishi eventually helped devise a program that would compress and rank every single player available. It was initially based on 80 variables, but the rankings were eventually reduced to five components – character, body-control, competitiveness, mental alertness, and strength and explosiveness. The computer model Qureishi devised has been credited for the team bringing in the likes of Mel Renfro, Bobby Hayes, Roger Staubach, Craig Morton, Jethro Pugh, Walt Garrison, Rayfield Wright, Larry Cole, Calvin Hill, and Duane Thomas.

In 1967, Murchison took this technology to create a new company called "Optimum Systems," which held the rights to the player-selection evaluation system created by Qureishi. The company was owned by the Cowboys, Rams, 49ers, Saints, and by the inventor himself.

When the Cowboys were considering a trade up to the Seattle Seahawks for a running back in the 1977 NFL Draft, the computer ranking system was clear – make the deal. A scout said, "I bow to the computer." The player was Pittsburgh running back Tony Dorsett, who eventually would be inducted to the Pro Football Hall of Fame. The computer program was not foolproof – the Cowboys still had dud draft picks just like every other team – but it reduced the margin for error and kept everybody organized.

"That was all Tex," Gil Brandt said. "We were really lucky to find [Qureishi]."

The odd pairing of the hard-driving Murchison – who was known to drink and party for hours – and the reserved Qureishi eventually dissolved. The latter left the team in 1972 to form his own company. Though he was long gone by the time Ward arrived to the Cowboys in 1976, everything he put into place was still there and in use. Qureishi briefly returned to the Cowboys in 1986, but by the time he came back, the NFL had caught up to his innovations and surpassed them. Nonetheless, when the team hired him, there was nobody else like him in professional sports.

Sort of like their hiring of Dr. Bob Ward.

• • • •

When Ward was offered the job, the team was in the midst of the second-most dominant run of any NFL team in that era. The only team that was more successful than the Cowboys was the Pittsburgh Steelers, who defeated the Cowboys twice in the Super Bowl in the '70s.

The Cowboys were the anti-Steelers with an established identity and a niche that endures to this day. The term, "America's Team" – coined by Schramm – remains one of the most copied, debated, yet undoubtedly successful monikers any team has had. The team embraced and embodied the professionalization of sports long before every other franchise in every other league.

The football team is one of the biggest reasons the city of Dallas eventually shed the image as the town where President John F. Kennedy was assassinated. The scars from that tragic event on November 22, 1963, lasted for years and became a national identity for Dallas. It was not until the football team, the growth of the American southwest, and eventually the wildly popular CBS TV show *Dallas* did the image and the reputation of the city began to change into a glitzy, sexy place to be – located halfway between Los Angeles and Miami.

When the Cowboys interviewed Ward in the spring of 1976, the team was coming off a 10-4 season and an NFC title. They had won road games in the playoffs – at Minnesota in the NFC divisional round in the famous "Hail Mary" pass from Roger Staubach to Drew Pearson for a game-winning touchdown on the game's final play. The Cowboys defeated the Los Angeles Rams in the NFC title game in Los Angeles to advance to the Super Bowl, where they were defeated by their nemesis, the Pittsburgh Steelers.

The Dallas Cowboys were already successful without Bob Ward. The Cowboys at that time were so good they were not going to implode without his arrival. The roster included Roger Staubach, Rayfield Wright, Ed "Too Tall" Jones, Harvey Martin, Mel Renfro, Charlie Waters, Cliff Harris, among many other notable football names from that era. They knew they had talent, but they also realized they needed someone to get more out of that talent.

"He was the right guy at the right time," Brandt said.

They wanted an updated version of Alvin Roy. The Cowboys wanted the strength training combined with the explosive speed and speed endurance training. That didn't mean the likes of Landry, Brandt, or Schramm knew the specifics, but they knew enough to know there was more out there to be had.

"We had Alvin Roy in that job before and what we wanted was somebody who was doing the kinds of research into endurance and strength," Brandt said. "We did want somebody different than Alvin. He was good; he would bring his track coach from LSU, Boots Garland, over to our facility three times a year to focus on running. And that was it. The running and endurance part of it was not something he was an expert in. We wanted to incorporate all of it. Alvin was a guy who would say, 'Give me 12 more sets of everything and I'll get you to the Olympics.'"

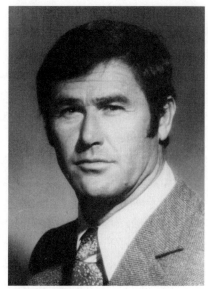

Bob Ward's team photo after he joined the Dallas Cowboys in 1976.

They didn't know much about Ward, other than he came highly recommended by the guy they wanted, who was the suggestion of the successful UCLA head football coach, Dick Vermeil. The Cowboys simply knew that Ward was at the front end of something that was coming, and they didn't want to be second.

"I never knew where Tom Landry found him," former Dallas Cowboys linebacker Thomas "Hollywood" Henderson said. "But I knew exactly why they hired him – he was revolutionary. As far as I am concerned, Bob Ward revolutionized training for football."

A revolution that began in 1976 when the Dallas Cowboys hired him.

Ward's Words
The Best Coaches

Over four decades, I had the pleasure of working with some of the very best coaches in sports, whether it was track or football. I can't possibly rank these men in order, but of the many men I was blessed to work with there was none any better than Tom Landry. The man was so ahead of his time, so smart and so analytical. People didn't know he could be malleable. He had this very calm presence, and he knew what everybody was doing and needed to do. He didn't show a lot in terms of emotion; he didn't show a lot at all. He was just an exceptional man.

Here are some of the other coaches I worked with who were some of the very best:

- *Tom Tellez, UCLA and Houston track and field coach. We were at Fullerton Community College together and he was just so smart. The man is so bright, and he was one of those guys who believed in research and analytics before so many other people did. He was an exceptional coach.*
- *Jim Myers, Dallas Cowboys offensive line coach. He did things that people would not do; a lot of guys did not like him because he would get in their face. He would chew them out. And he did not back down from anybody. He would do things for Coach Landry that he would not do for anyone.*
- *Gene Stallings, Cowboys assistant coach. Gene was an old-school coach and he didn't necessarily believe in all of the things that I did with the Cowboys, but he never got in the way. What was so shocking about Gene is that he was quiet and stoic, but the minute he needed be in front of a crowd or an*

audience, he was a brilliant, silver-tongued speaker. I'll never get over how quiet he was because the minute you put him front of a room full of people, he could talk and stir people up in a way that you didn't recognize him. He is a good Christian man who was so good to me and my family.

- *Dan Reeves, Cowboys assistant coach. A great man. Dan was one of these guys, like a lot of us, who was really shaped by Coach Landry. Of all the guys I worked with, it looked like Dan tried to be the most like Tom. He too was very stoic, very calm, and you were going to do things his way.*

- *Mike Ditka, Cowboys assistant coach. A total in your face guy; he was a former player, but he had the professional experience and he did not back down. We were playing Atlanta, and somebody knocked receiver Drew Pearson over the bench on our sidelines. So, Ditka instinctively went over and punched the Falcons player as a way to defend our players against any further blows. He had a good practical way about him, protective. He was like Jim Myers in that way.*

- *Vince Lombardi, New York Giants assistant coach. He was just excellent. All of these guys in that era, whether it was with the Giants or later with the Cowboys, they all had military backgrounds; that's what Vince had. He was no-nonsense, and just remarkably well organized, and knew how to coach people as well as anyone ever has.*

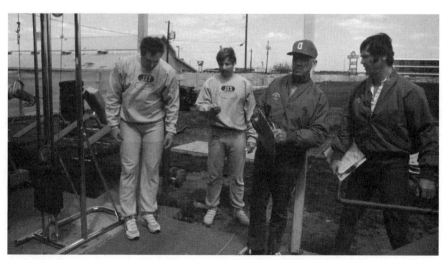

Longtime Dallas Cowboys assistant coach Jim Myers (middle) and Bob Ward at the team's facility in Dallas. Myers was a trusted confidant of Tom Landry and a close friend to Ward. Bob Ward spoke at Jim Myers' funeral.

CHAPTER 5

PREDICTIONS

*"The future belongs to those who see possibilities before
they become obvious."*
– John Sculley, former CEO of Apple

Sports is loaded with bright thinkers and a far greater number of people whose intellectual capacity is never fully fleshed out. These people are more commonly called "dummies." There are your random dummies, and then there are those who simply learned enough of the peripheral as a means to advance in their chosen fields. Most people in sports dedicate the majority of their time to improving their bodies and their physical abilities. Education, to the majority of people who "make it" in sports, is not the priority as much as performance; it becomes secondary. When the athlete retires, they often continue in the profession either as a coach, teacher, scout, or executive. A great many of them never complete college, so they maybe never pushed their intellectual capabilities beyond their chosen field because they didn't want to or they did not have to.

This does not mean the jock is dumb or the retired athlete is an idiot incapable of doing anything more than playing ball. Quite the contrary; to be truly successful in an industry as savage as pro sports, one cannot be stupid. Eventually, the brain has to do *something*. Maybe the athlete will never qualify to teach at Yale or do extensive research at NASA, but in their chosen field, they have to be smart enough to figure out how to thrive, or at least survive.

What made Bob Ward stand out, especially in the '70s and '80s, was that he was in a professional society that, at that point, still did not place value on higher education the way it does now. In the '70s, pro football was football. Sports was mostly *just* sports. It was a business, sure, but not to the extent that it is today.

Most strength and conditioning coaches have a background beyond the weight room, and they usually at some point played at a higher level. You don't find a lot of ex-golfers, swimmers, tennis, baseball, or basketball players creating a second career in the field of strength and conditioning coaches; they are or were more often football players or track guys. These are guys who love lifting and fitness.

In 1976, a strength or conditioning coach in professional sports who had a doctorate, such as Dr. Bob Ward, was the ultimate outlier.

Since then, sports has become a multi-billion dollar business that has drawn and inspired forward and revolutionary thinking all in the name of defeating an opponent in a game. A strength coach with a PED is not common, but it's now not entirely uncommon.

A football trainer likened talking to Bob Ward to a maze. Former football player Kevin Callaway, who spent one offseason with the Dallas Cowboys in 1984, called Ward "an absolute genius."

Ward is not Nostradamus, but in professional sports, he did see things that not just anyone could have predicted. Former USC All-American shot putter Dave Murphy, who worked with Ward in high school and at Fullerton Community College in the late '60s, said: "He was a little bit ahead of the Russian scientists."

In the summer of 1982, Bob Ward had long since earned his doctorate from Indiana University and was entrenched as a staff member of the Dallas Cowboys. His status as the conditioning coach of America's Team granted him access pretty much anywhere he wanted in sports, and he opened his doors to anybody who wanted to see what he was doing. In his field, he was a celebrity and a scientist, and science, at its core, is about a freedom of information.

The Cold War was still a few years away from its conclusion, and ESPN was still a long way away from forever changing the direction of professional sports. The power player in technology was IBM even though personal laptops had not yet been created. Steve Jobs was still trying to figure out how to improve and market his "Macintosh" computer. In 1980, Bill Gates and Paul Allen formed a startup company called "Microsoft" and were approaching the day when they would release "Windows" to the world.

By 1982, after working and studying with United States Olympic teams, Ward had enough experience to know that the sports we all knew in the 20th century would look vastly different in the 21st century. He had seen enough to recognize that sports, and people's infinite desire to win or improve, would be vastly changed thanks to technology. He had worked and trained enough to predict that what was coming in sports was going to be a competitive fight for every single advantage available, and the amount of money pouring in made it lucrative for bright people to make it their career.

· · · ·

In the June-July 1982 edition of the *National Strength and Conditioning Association Journal*, Ward wrote an article called "Superconditioning Technologies For Sports in the Twenty-first Century." Few sports fans would have ever read this article. Even for those who did read it in 1982, few could have believed what he wrote would not only happen, but would happen soon. As a rule of thumb, smart people see what's coming before it actually happens, which is exactly what Ward did.

This is a three-page study that essentially predicts the future of sports with an almost prophetic accuracy. Based on his previous experiences, studies, and projections, what Bob Ward wrote in the summer of 1982 is so freakishly accurate in many areas that he would have been wiser to take his talents to Las Vegas or the stock market and go heavy into futures. What begins as a fairly benign piece about the future of sports training eventually goes places that only a few might have predicted.

Ward writes in his introduction:

> "Very few programs develop out of thin air. ... So, it is vital to be receptive to unknown or unfamiliar ideas of the past, present, and future; if not, we too often dismiss old ideas and theories as outdated, present methods as either risky or absolute, and future concepts as unattainable, impractical or too way out. With this attitude, new insights are few.
> "Mishima, a Japanese writer, aptly advises of the weakness of finding truth in that way when he said: 'There are some truths in this world that one cannot see unless one unbends one's posture.' – Sun and Steel"

In this article, Ward articulates principles that were nearly all rooted in the concept that "everything affects everything"; nothing is truly separate. Anything a person does in the name of improvement can impact them positively in a number of different areas of their lives. Ward preached the totality of everything in the name of improvement. That sport is not just about ball, bat, stick, glove, shot put, or discus but rather the evolution of movement and seeking of improvement in mind and body.

Ward's predictions of the modern day athlete and their improvement is like the opening sequence of Stanley Kubrick's sci-fi classic film *2001:*

A Space Odyssey. Made in 1968, the opening scene of the movie involves a primitive landscape where apes roam around in what appears to be the dawn of man; one ape grabs a bone, and in one fluid, slow-motion, the white bone floats down through the sky and morphs into a space ship floating through the silence of deep space. The obvious conclusion is this is how primitive man began and where he has gone.

Ward views the origins of a Tom Brady pass or a LeBron James dunk not in Roger Staubach or Michael Jordan but rather the first human beings who ran, lifted a heavy object, or threw something. The goal has been to improve the efficiency with which we perform those physical tasks, and it all begins in the movement of the mind to the body.

The introduction continues:

> "Hopefully in the course of this discussion you will begin to see that there is a movement in our country founded on the desire to seek better solutions to old problems for attaining higher levels of performance. This movement is having an impact right now, and it will have an even greater impact in the future. …
>
> "… Ironically, many of you will recognize some of these methods for the future because they have been part of your program in the past. There is a good reason to believe that many of the methods that man has used for survival and sport have been with us from the beginning of time. Many of the methods have been lost, then rediscovered by some future age. Old or new, they still weave their magic on the performance of those who adhere to the essence of their principles. Everyone of us has that built-in element of creative genius which allows us to surpass our own expectations and those of people around us. … The only criterion we require for evaluating our course is that whatever we do must be a 'Reflection of Reality.'"

What Ward believed then is now widely accepted as fact: "It's a total holistic approach," Houston Astros strength and conditioning coach Jake Beiting said. For the record, Beiting has never met Ward, but he unknowingly uses one of the Ward's buzz words – holistic - when it comes to preparation and performance enhancement. "It's not just lifting weight – what goes into a guy physically to be ready to play every day?" Beiting said. "It's every single thing they do."

What Dr. Bob Ward wrote three decades ago resonates loudly with the current state of competitive sports.

• • • •

SPORT

"Many people have seen the same or similar visionary processes required for developing and maintaining unusual levels of performance. Similarly, any program must have a vision of the goal it seeks. It is absolutely essential in any High Performance Conditioning Program. One of the best statements I have ever read was written by Bruce Lee. In his model, 'Competition' is the focal point of the discussion. However, I feel that the concept can and should be extended to any aspect of living. Lee states, 'Competition "as is" is total, and it includes all that "is" as well as "is not," without favorite lines or angles. Lacking boundaries, competition is always fresh, alive and constantly changing. Your particular style, your personal inclinations and your physical makeup are all parts of competition, but they do not constitute the whole of competition. Should your responses become dependent upon any single part, you will react in terms of "what should be" rather than to the reality of the everchanging "what is." Remember that while the whole is evident in all its parts, an isolated part efficient or not, does not constitute the whole.'"

Ward stressed the willingness to adapt, to be flexible, and to always remain open minded. For all of its evolution, sports can be rooted in the realities of tradition. Change is not easily accepted by anybody, even with the incentive to find or create a different way. Player training and player evaluation, two key components to success in sports, should – in theory – always be rapidly evolving. But, even now, these areas face the innate challenges of change. Doing things differently from the way they have always been done is forever difficult.

TECHNOLOGY COMPUTERIZES THE GAME

The computer technology of 30 years ago was almost nothing compared to its omnipresence today. Cell phones, for the most part, did not exist. Email was not a part of the international lexicon – yet. Email has existed since 1965, most likely beginning at the Massachusetts Institute of Technology (MIT). It slowly started to grow and was something Bob Ward was using in the '70s when he worked with the United States Olympic program. He was one of the few who had access to that then small piece of technology; as such, he could see that this was a trend that would only grow and eventually revolutionize nearly every society in the world. By 1982, Ward was already well immersed in using computers to analyze and measure athletes and prescribe computerized conditioning programs. He could see some of the global electronic revolution coming because he was on the front lines to a certain degree.

"Technology will be so powerful that elements of the actual game can be recorded with great precision. Analysis of this game data will confirm that intuitively initiated behavior is a sound method for decision making. In fact, the difference between levels of performance may well be described on a scale designated for measuring instantaneous apprehension, and action of players. Therefore, a great amount of effort will be spent exploring Psycho/Physical domain. However, don't think that this exploration will be limited to the esoteric or mystical areas at the expense of training and the understanding of our sensory systems. It may be that the most startling discoveries will come from the apparently familiar."

Cut through it, and what Ward explains is exactly what has happened – sports rely on computers as much as any other business or facet of modern society in the 21st century. NFL teams now use iPads on the sidelines to review plays, formations, etc., and they're not alone. All MLB, NHL

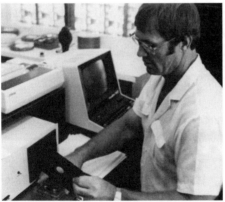

and NBA teams are immersed in data. What Ward was doing with technology and computers in the '70s with the Cowboys, *everybody* has come to embrace in sports. Today, there is hardly a single sports act left unaffected or undocumented by computers and technology.

Here is Bob Ward working on one of those computers in 1977 at the Cowboys' team facility in Dallas. Although he didn't introduce computers to the Dallas Cowboys, Ward allowed them to capitalize on technology when its use was still uncommon in the NFL.

What is now a commonly-used and widely-practiced noun – "analytics" – was made possible through the types of measurements Ward developed during his career.

Ward envisioned a world that combined split-second breakdowns, made possible by science and computers, with a deep exploration of the human mind. Psychology is a major portion of the sports landscape today.

PSYCHO/PHYSICAL

Ward was born in 1933, the son of a World War I veteran, and down the street from a factory that produced airplanes that dropped bombs in World War II. He was a Marine between the United States' military campaigns in Korea and Vietnam. He lived through the Cold War when paranoia was rampant and spying was routine. There was zero cooperation between the United States and the then U.S.S.R.

During the Cold War, the Soviets and other Eastern Bloc countries thrived in certain sports and were on the same level as the Americans in terms of athletic training. But there had not been an open exchange of information between the two sides.

"It was so hard to get information from Russia, or any Soviet country, because it was the Cold War," Dave Murphy said. "I do remember when we would face the U.S.S.R. in certain meets and they would always have interpreters with them. It was all very hush-hush what they would talk about, and answer. We would learn some things, but not very much."

Both sides were testing and going places in sports science without the benefit of the other's direct knowledge. It was like the Space Race – the U.S.S.R. did its thing, as did the U.S. It was a competition of athletes and scientists. No one knew exactly what those Eastern Bloc methods were, but everyone saw how well their ways worked during the international competitions, where they thrived. Specifically, Eastern Bloc countries such as Hungary, Poland, Russia, Belarus, Estonia, and Communist Cuba all dominated weightlifting during the Cold War. They had good athletes, but they also had good training methods as well as wonderful doctors and scientists. In the early '80s, however, it was widely known that the Soviets and other Eastern Bloc countries had been using steroids and other synthetic means to better their athletes.

"Eastern and western thought will form a comprehensive system in which there will be no differentiation between east or west. Rather, a *multidimensional* blend will emerge to form a global/holistic system – one that includes many factors. Western science will confirm the value of using intuitive systems of information processing. This concept will reconfirm the Greek concept of Mind and Body – a Unity – Inseparable. Fantastic new breakthroughs will be made in understanding how the body functions as an integrated whole. Again, the psychosomatic idea enters on the scene to re-establish its reign."

Ward was wise enough to know the Cold War would not last forever, which would allow for scientists in the field of sports to do what most scientists do – exchange ideas and information. When this article was published, the U.S. had already boycotted the 1980 Summer Olympic Games in Moscow in large part as a protest of the Soviets' invasion of Afghanistan.

In 1982, and during the next several years, the idea of the East and West embracing each other with peace, or an exchange of ideas via a means that were not stolen, was highly improbable. Ward had an idea it would happen eventually.

In 1989, Communism officially fell, and Ward's vision of exchanging ideas and concepts did indeed happen. The two sides that were once bitter enemies today share a space station together for one reason – science.

Brian Weese has been a professional athletic trainer at Texas Tech University for six and a half years, and now works with football players preparing for the NFL Draft. He's worked with USA Track and Field, USA Weightlifting, and is a Certified Speed & Explosion Specialist with many additional certifications to his name. He said, "Dr. Ward was doing this before this was a profession, and he knew about this before Eastern Bloc methods and training... he was right there in the mix of what it was evolving into and becoming. He went head to head against the Russians, the Bulgarians and saw what they were doing was better than what everybody else was doing.

"And what we have learned, today, is that after all of the changes and fads that our profession has gone through, really since the '90s, is that the way Dr. Ward operated and the Eastern Bloc method is still the best way."

SUPER LEARNING CENTERS

"Traditional classroom environments will be dramatically changed into 'Star Wars'- like settings. Every athlete is made an active part of the learning process. No one can hide. Electronic systems become inter-locked with the athlete/instructor/material to form an open/closed circuit. The clarity of data or information transmission defies all explanations. Little doubt will be left in the information system because concrete methods are used over abstract methods. The knowledge of results is instantaneously recognized within the complexity of the task. Difficult tasks will come closer to sports such as archery, where proficiency is known instantly."

This comes back to technology. There is almost nothing wrong or inaccurate about Ward's vision of "Super Learning Centers." Information systems are in real-time and available for nearly everybody with a computer and access to the Internet. And forget archery – instantaneous access is available to NBA, NFL, NHL and MLB teams in a way that was simply inconceivable in 1982.

BIOFEEDBACK

"Biofeedback instrumentation will be utilized to help the athlete assume a state of awareness essential to performance at high levels of skill. Although biofeedback methods may assist positively in the process of training, self-development procedures will prove to be the desired methods. In this regard, the Zen concept of total awareness also may be the objective sought via the biofeedback method. Many athletes who previously had little hope of reaching higher levels of awareness will be able to attain higher levels of awareness that will enhance performance. Other multi-sensory technologies already seeing limited use will be commonplace in tomorrow's training facility."

Today, nearly every single athlete of every variety can receive Biofeedback on their phone, their watch, and in nearly every single gym in America. By the definition of the Mayo Clinic, biofeedback is a technique that you can use "to learn to control your body's functions, such as your heart rate." The whole concept is rooted in the idea that you can use your thoughts to control your body.

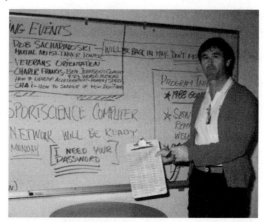

Bob Ward would write extensive notes on his "workout board" at the team's practice facility in Valley Ranch. He may not have had a "Super Learning Center," but Ward was always sharing what he knew with players and other coaches.

SENSORY ISOLATION TANKS

"Sensory isolation tanks will be a common training tool in the twenty-first century learning center. These tanks systematically reduce sensory input to levels that reduce the energy requirements for relaxation. These tank systems will be equipped with highly sophisticated, computer driven biofeedback and sensory enhancing devices to provide a multi-sensory learning mechanism of high impact."

In 2015, a sensory isolation tank is also called a "float spa." These small compartments have become increasingly popular among the wealthier crowd looking to "float" and relax. A person sits, or "floats" in a approximately 10 inches of water and more than 1,000 pounds of Epsom salt, that is heated to about 95 degrees. This process is called "flotation therapy," and it is becoming more widely used. The experience is billed as a rejuvenation and relaxation of the mind and body.

In this same strata is cryotherapy – a moderately popular means of relaxation but more known as a means of accelerated healing. The Vancouver Canucks NHL team used this in the mid-'90s; the subzero temperatures used in these pods are designed to decrease inflammation, pain, spasms, etc. while increasing cellular survival.

Whether or not these means of improvement work depends on the individual athlete.

HOLOGRAPHIC PROJECTION

"Holographic methods will help close the gap between any simulated and actual skill. This technique will use state-of-the-art laser technology to project any kind of action in three-dimensional space (projected into thin air). Imagine the situation: a wide receiver that you have to cover in the next game actually at your facility running untiringly, all of his favorite routes for you to cover. ... Holography is a step closer to that reality, but it can never take the place of the actual situation itself."

Sounds a bit like a *Madden NFL* EA Sports video game, but in terms of a New York Giants receiver like Odell Beckham Jr. practicing against a holographic 3-D image of Pro Football Hall of Fame cornerback Deion Sanders, it has not happened yet. Simulations featuring computer imagery of players, golf courses, mountains and terrains have all happened. Companies will pay big money to athletes and cover the sensory-gathering technology in an effort to build road maps to their movements, but in terms of 1-on-1 preparation, that is a feat that's not quite there.

Virtual reality technology developed by former Stanford University kicker Derek Belch and StriVR Labs is being used at several major college programs, including Arkansas, Clemson, Vanderbilt, and Auburn.

In the spring of 2015, the Dallas Cowboys added a virtual reality component to their facilities. The team built a sound-proof room where players sit down and put on a headset. The player can then see a full 360-degree shot of the practice, downloaded onto the headset. In the NFL, where normally the people who practice during the week are the starters, this technology is invaluable to backups. It allows a player to see the same play repeatedly from every possible angle.

"You can rewind it as many times as you want and really get a grasp of fine tuning each play," Dallas Cowboys veteran backup quarterback Brandon Weeden said. "Out there [on the field] it happens so fast, you're kind of running plays, and it's rapid fire. In there, it gives you the ability to rewind it, really understand it."

PERSONALITY ASSESSMENT

In 1982, the first pick in the NFL Draft by the New England Patriots was a defensive end from the University of Texas named Kenneth Sims. That same year, the Los Angeles Lakers selected North Carolina forward James Worthy with the first overall pick of a draft that then had 10 rounds. It is safe to say neither of these men had to endure anything compared to the No. 1 overall pick in any major sports league today.

"Personality assessment tools of the future will become more refined and will provide the player, and coach, with an opportunity to know themselves and each other more completely."

Franchises spend hundreds of thousands of dollars in an effort to figure out what a player's mind is like and use every tool available to see if a potential acquisition has the necessary mental capacity. It is not uncommon for teams, usually those of the NFL, to hire investigators to research a player's background as well.

In 2014, the Boston Celtics were exploring the possibility of selecting Oklahoma State guard Marcus Smart in the upcoming NBA Draft. In an effort to find out everything they could about Smart, Celtics general manager Danny Ainge told *The Boston Globe*, "Sometimes we dig as deep as talking to a player's high school teachers and college professors. Suffice it to say we talked to dozens of people that were close to Marcus."

This is not an exception but the rule, as is the standard of nearly every team having a psychologist on its payroll.

In terms of mental testing, one of the more common tools NFL teams now use is the Wonderlic test; it can be used to estimate a player's IQ and aptitude for learning and, more specifically, problem solving. Players have 12 minutes to answer 50 questions that evaluate reasoning skills. Now, whether the team actually uses these tests is a different matter. The national average for correct answers is 22; chemists, for example, score 31.

Some teams use the test as a "tie breaker" of sorts. If the team has the choice between two players of equal athletic prowess, the "smarter" guy is typically selected. In 1986, *The Florida Times Union* and the *St. Petersburg Times* obtained the Wonderlic test results of all the first round draft picks that year.

The highest score for all first rounders that year was 34, by Virginia offensive lineman Jim Dombrowski. He played 11 productive seasons with the New Orleans Saints. The lowest reported score was 13, by four players, including Oklahoma defensive tackle Tony Casillas. Casillas was selected with the second pick by the Atlanta Falcons; in 12 NFL seasons, he played for three teams and won a Super Bowl with the Dallas Cowboys. He was a nice player, but if you talked to him and saw what he did with his post-NFL life – where he has carved out a successful career in broadcasting – the test result doesn't do justice to his professional success.

By the way, the player who went first in that draft scored a 17 on the test. His name was Bo Jackson, one of the greatest athletes of any generation. Bo knew a lot, including that some tests just don't matter if you're Bo Jackson.

There are instances, of course, when the test is the reddest of red flags. For example, in the 2012 NFL Draft, LSU cornerback Morris Claiborne reportedly put up the lowest score ever recorded by an athlete on an official NFL Wonderlic test. He finished with a 4. But, because he rated so highly in athletics – speed, agility, jumping, hands – the Dallas Cowboys selected

Claiborne with the sixth pick in that draft anyway.

The tools to measure and assess personality are there and are frequently used. Whether or not they are applied is situational or more often based on convenience.

"Most teams discuss character," said the former general manager of the Texas Rangers, Tom Grieve. "But what happens is in composite. You look beyond what you know is best and disregard enough evidence to take a chance on a guy because he's so talented."

SUPER INTELLIGENCE

"Super Intelligence is concerned with the individual or collective processing of information. Any member of the sports team will be able to use the information processing of this highly sophisticated computer network to answer any question. In organizations requiring security, the system will have its own unique structure. However, it will resemble the free network of people who are linked together philosophically, and also physically, for the purpose of improving performance. For instance, a member of the network may have a conditioning problem requiring expert advice. All one needs to do is get on the computerized teleconferencing network and the answers from the expert members of the network will be on the computer in a minimum amount of time. Network problem solving will provide expert consensus never before enjoyed to quickly solve pressing problems."

This concept of integrated and real-time problem solving technology is now applied to nearly every major business, school, and medical facility. It has also revolutionized how companies conduct customer service where people routinely go to the Internet to find answers from experts who are sitting at their computer ready to help.

EDUCATIONAL NETWORKS

"Professional education networks will change the traditional ways of certifying students and teaching courses. Selection of instructors can be made from some of the best minds in the areas of your interests. The impact will cross all levels of education including undergraduate, graduate, and continuing education. A system such as this can only lead to greater professional excellence."

Much like every other facet of society, education is now a giant business that creates certifications, degrees, licenses, etc. in nearly every field including sports training, sports science, sports psychology, etc.

BIOMECHANICS

"Biomechanics is a scientific technology lurking in the background as a super spy. More and more information is being presented today using this remarkable body of knowledge, interfaced with computer technology. Most of the impact has been in skill analysis and improvement in various items of equipment. In the twenty-first century, it will be firmly implanted into all aspects of sport. Games with opponents can be programmed to be played prior to the actual game with data that is collected from previous contests. Game plans and strategies based on this process surely will bring a Super Intelligence program to the field on the day of the game. Trends and patterns of play will be immediately discernable and thereby initiate immediate counter-actions from participants."

This area has transformed Major League Baseball, some would argue not for the better, and nearly every other aspect of mid or high major sports. Statistics have always existed in sport, but since Ward wrote this article, the amount of computer analysis has increased at a rate that would seem impossible back then. Data analysis – go ahead and call it "analytics" – has completely changed the way teams treat their players and games.

A big league baseball manager can have, nearly instantly, every at bat and every result in nearly every possible scenario at his fingertips for the batter who is in the on deck circle. This sort of analysis can be overkill, but it has created ways and means to produce a more efficient player. There is no correlation between success and more numbers, but there is a direct linkage between the winner and those who have found the *meaning* in the numbers.

Just tracking the number of pitches thrown by a major league pitcher has transformed the way pitchers are treated, evaluated, and graded. It was not until the late '80s that teams began to count the number of pitches thrown by pitchers.

In 1988, Nolan Ryan started 33 games for the Houston Astros. Only six times did he fail to throw 100 pitches. He was 41 years old. He was 12-11 that season with a 3.52 ERA.

In 2012, Johnny Cueto started 33 games for the Cincinnati Reds. Twelve times he did not hit 100 pitches in a game. He was 26 years old. He finished the season 19-9 with a 2.78 earned run average, and led the National League in starts, and finished fourth in the NL Cy Young voting as the league's best overall pitcher.

Since teams began to count the number of pitches thrown, they quickly discovered a direct link between the number of pitches thrown and effectiveness. The more a pitcher pitches, the less effective he generally becomes. That's why starting pitchers seldom throw 110 pitches any more.

In the '80s, before this type of research was done, there were signs it was coming.

"When Nolan Ryan was with the [California] Angels, he typically threw about 180 pitches per game," Dr. Gene Coleman said, who directed conditioning for the Astros when Ryan, a 33-year-old veteran, left the Angels to sign with Houston in 1980. "A bad game for him was 212 pitches. I think he went up to 235 pitches in a 13-inning game once.

"By the time he was around 30, he could not get into the eighth or ninth inning. When he was with the Angels, if he got into the eighth or ninth he never lost. For us, if he hit 155 pitches, he was topping out. And he was pushing it if he got there. We would keep track of his pitches on 3-2 [counts]. Nolan's thing was, 'If I get to 3-2, it's over' [implying he would get the hitter out]. Typically, a pitcher throws five pitches in 3-2 counts. Nolan was going to eight pitches on 3-2. That means he was throwing 64 pitches to eight batters. And we found he was not striking everybody out. About 60 percent of the guys he faced on 3-2 were getting on base. He would say, 'On 3-2, I'm not adjusting.' It's the 'I'm the Fastest Gun in the West' mentality.

"So if he would not change how he would throw on 3-2, he would on 2-2. He changed how he pitched on 2-2 counts, and he cut his numbers from throwing 64 pitches to 32 pitches, and that enabled us to get him into the eighth and ninth inning."

Now apply this same type of analytical approach to every player in every sport. The efficiency has increased exponentially since 1982.

Of the many areas Ward predicted for the 21st century, the following is perhaps most remarkable:

SUPER BOWL – TWENTY FIRST CENTURY

"Let's see if we can imagine a twenty-first century international Super Bowl between the Russian Bears, winner of the eastern hemisphere conference championship game, and the western hemisphere's representative, the American Cowboys. Some of the innovations we will see during the game could possibly be:

Playing environment

— Completely controlled

— Playing surface ideal for safety and play

— Biochemically designed surfaces designed to spread the force of impact over time and even improve running speed

Space Age Uniforms

— Biochemically designed to protect the body and still provide tremendous comfort.

— Physiologically instrumented for monitoring all systems.

Skills of the Players

— Biomechanically improved for maximum performance.

— Martial arts training aiding the players in achieving new levels of excellence in their skills.

Pattern Analysis of the Game

— Biomechanical and computer technology merge to give precise movement patterns of all players and plays. Once in the computer, the visual replay on the screen can be rotated to any view desired (top/side/rear).

— Forces of impact will be displayed along with the velocities and accelerations of players, and the ball in kicking and passing.

— Officiating will move into the twenty-first century, also. The officiating system will include all of the biomechanical-computer capabilities used to analyze the game plus other unique sub-systems. Each official will wear instrumentation showing the field of his visual focus. This data will be stored on tape and be available for evaluation in controversial situations. The position of the football will be determined biomechanically by using multi-television cameras. The football will also be equipped with microelectronics to assist in determining its position on the field.

Complete historical data from all previous contests will be available for a variety of uses.

— Compare and recap plays.
— Predict play selection.
— Predict game winner.
— Statistical reports.

Spectators will interact in the game, not only as fans but also as active armchair coaches. All stadium seats will be electronically wired for consensus voting. The results of such opinions will use electronic scoreboards for reporting results. This will lead, of course, to greater spectator involvement."

Ward wrote these predictions in 1982 when dome stadiums were at a relative infancy – there were five NFL teams that played in controlled environments. By 2014, the figure doubled to 10.

AstroTurf, which by the '80s was the common surface for football stadiums at both the professional and college level, has been deemed archaic and cruel to the human body. Most teams now use a "sports surface" – a synthetic that is easier on the bones and still allows for a better grip and speed. It's not grass, but it's certainly not the painful concrete-like surface that was AstroTurf.

Equipment and uniforms are now continually updated and scientifically studied to be lighter, to reduce water quicker, and to fit better. Sometimes, these improvements are made in the name of performance; in others, these improvements are made for the sake of increasing profits for companies such as Nike, Reebok, Under Armour, etc.

Players now routinely participate in other forms of exercise in the name of more strength, or flexibility. Yoga, martial arts, boxing, etc. are alternative forms of exercise players now try, and no one thinks twice about using them. Ward was one of the very first to do this, as his players embraced quick-striking and rapid-movement exercises, namely martial arts based on Bruce Lee's – and Lee-trainee, Dan Inosanto's – martial arts systems.

On telecasts, networks routinely show viewers how fast something is moving, whether it be the receiver or the flight of the ball. In telecasts of MLB games, fans now always have access to the radar gun to see how fast pitches travel to home plate. The power of impact, however, is something "still missing."

Officials in all sports are now constantly scrutinized, judged, and graded based on data analysis. They are monitored for everything, from the number of pass interference penalties called in a certain game, down to the record of the road teams in the playoff game when a particular referee is calling a game.

Retired Pro Football Hall of Fame NFL football coach Bill Parcells was renowned for tracking officials; he would closely monitor who was working his team's upcoming game and adjust accordingly. In the NBA, certain officials have reputations for calling certain fouls, and since Ward wrote this article, anything a referee does can easily be quantified and researched.

As of early 2014, tennis was on the verge of being able to eliminate humans from "calling games." The "Hawk-Eye" lines-calling system has been in tennis for about a decade, and one series – the PowerShares Series – eliminated line judges altogether to, instead, rely on the players to call in or out and, should it be necessary, the "Hawk-Eye" replay.

In terms of the statistical analysis available, smartphones have revolutionized what fans can access and track during the game. In 1982, a fan had to wait for statistics to be displayed on a monitor or scoreboard at the game or wait for the public address announcer to read them. Now, with a smartphone, a fan can track any stat from any game in real time.

SUPER NUTRITION

"Biochemistry in the twenty-first century will provide the nutritional knowledge and products necessary for Super Adaptation of the body. Twentieth century nutrition will climb out of the dark ages, and turn into an age of greater awareness. We have known for years that there must be a balance between work, rest, and nutrition if performance levels are to be raised significantly. However, when each cell is provided with all of the nourishment it needs from Super Nutrition for power growth and functioning, remarkable changes will occur.

- Some of the common side effects of training, such as simple soreness, will be evident but at insignificant levels.
- Productive athlete years will be increased in the same proportions as the life expectancy increases to 120 years or more."

In Ward's tenure with the Cowboys, it was not uncommon for coaches in other sports to be highly selective of when their players could have water. There was a time when athletes were simply not given or allowed to have any. Water breaks were a treat, one often reserved for the weak. Now, virtually every doctor and professional attached to nutrition all agree – to hold back water from an athlete in training, who is burning calories and requires constant hydration, is inhumane.

Athletes are keenly aware of everything they put in their bodies these days, and trainers and teams alike spend countless hours and resources ensuring their cash cows are not loading up on junk. It is why when a professional athlete who tests positive for performance-enhancing drugs tries to explain it away as "I didn't know what I was taking," it's difficult to believe.

Teams will spend millions of dollars providing food – at nearly all hours – to the athletes to make sure their employees, their money-makers, are properly fueled. Nutrition has not always traveled at the same rate of technology since Ward wrote this study. Food is not just food, and calories are not just calories.

"I was with the Astros since the mid-'70s, and it was not until [pitcher] Roger Clemens and [pitcher] Andy Pettite got there from the Yankees did we have breakfast in the clubhouse," long time conditioning coach Dr. Gene Coleman said. "It was just some cereal and other stuff."

When Clemens and Pettite arrived after long careers with the highly successful New York Yankees, they *both* told the Astros they needed to have real breakfast available on game days. Food is important, but it wasn't to the Astros when Clemens and Pettite arrived; one of the oldest truisms in sports is doing everything the winner does in an effort to duplicate the results. The Astros started providing breakfast on game days soon after.

And there is such a thing as good fat. When outfielder Chad Curtis went to the Texas Rangers from the New York Yankees in 2000, he told the team the Yankees had junk food available. The point being, players needed to have at least a little bit of "give" to their bodies; that being built like a bronze

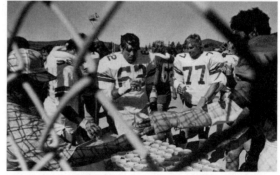

The Dallas Cowboys during a water break at training camp in the '70s. There was a time when athletes were simply not given or allowed to have water. Bob Ward emphasized the necessity of hydration shortly after he arrived to the team in 1976.

statue was not necessarily in the best interests of playing a brutal 162-game schedule. Again, do as the winner does.

About the only thing here Ward really whiffed on is life expectancy. No one is living 120 years – although there are many more living past 100 or even 110 than there used to be. According to The World Bank, in 1982, the average life expectancy for an American was 74 years; as late as 2015, it was up to 79 years. So, perhaps by the end of the 21st century, we will be up to the 120 years Ward projected.

TRADITIONAL PROGRAMS

"Many elements of the traditional programs will be found in the twenty-first century. The major difference will be that the exercises will be performed on devices capable of measuring the work done in a unified energy unit. The ability to place all sorts of exercises on the same scale will certainly aid in development of individual programs, as well as provide a means of evaluating all aspects of the exercise program.

"Global exercise programs will be the predominant method used in high performance sports programs. A global program is one that includes all kinds of exercises that not only work many joints simultaneously, but also exercise the complete joint potential."

Not only does what athletes do today far exceed anything they were doing in the '50s and '60s, but the "complete body workout" is something that is pounded into the head of everyone who walks into a gym. If you workout the stomach, you must workout the back. If you do one side, you must work the other, etc. Keeping the body in balance is paramount.

Trainers, strength coaches, and nutritionists all agree that workout programs and regimens cannot be a one-size fits all design; a program needs to be tailored and structured to the individual's needs and body.

• • • •

When Dr. Bob Ward authored this article in 1982, some of what he wrote was beginning to happen, but the rapid ascent and marriage of money, time, and technology was years away. More than 25 years later, the accuracy of his predictions demonstrates his vast level of expertise in his field. He not only foresaw the revolution coming in strength and conditioning, but with the Cowboys, he actually catalyzed it.

CHAPTER 6

IMPROVING THE DALLAS COWBOYS

"Your assumptions are your windows on the world. Scrub them off every once in a while, or the light won't come in."
– Isaac Asimov

Bob Ward walked on to the practice field at the team headquarters of the Dallas Cowboys in early summer of 1976 with Mike Ditka to the type of day with which he was completely unfamiliar. A Californian, Ward believed the type of hot, humid, sunny days he suffered during his time in the Marines in Quantico, Virginia were hellish and unfair. Dallas, from June often through the end of September, can be an unrelenting oven of heat, pain, sweat, and uncomfortability. It can be so hot that the trees seem to sweat, and pools often are no relief. Anybody who arrives in Texas during the summer months as a new resident is often unprepared and easily dispirited by a searing heat that Texans wear like a Purple Heart. "You think this is hot?" they will ask in an effort to show you that 103 degrees, to them, is a cold front. This type of pointless heat was something Ward had never lived in before.

Ditka was an assistant coach under Tom Landry in 1976. He was showing Ward around the headquarters and pointed the new conditioning coach to his "office," which wasn't an office at all. It was the "Weight Area, Football Field, Locker Room Area."

The practice field was a mostly non-descript area off of Forest and Abrams Avenue in Dallas that featured a Tornado-style fence that fans could easily see through. A Pizza Hut was on one side of the field, and the balcony of the second floor of the Days Inn offered wonderful viewing of Cowboys practices. This Days Inn was often the hotel of choice for the Cowboys to house potential players and guests. Coincidentally, it provided a great chance for scouts from opposing teams to rent a room for the night and wake up in the morning to take notes on the Cowboys' practices. Whatever they were writing down and reporting back to their respective teams obviously didn't work – the Cowboys were one of the best teams of this era, using this facility that was basically like a giant zoo where the players were the pandas and the coaches were the keepers, all easily seen by an adoring or curious public. Cowboys personnel did patrol the area during crucial practices to ensure no spying, but nothing like the secretive and paranoid techniques college and pro teams use today.

Since this was the dead of the offseason, Ward began his leave of absence from Fullerton Community College. By that time, the Cowboys were one of the few teams that offered incentives to stick around town to condition and train in the offseason – $50 per optional workout.

"They did? Nobody ever paid me," quarterback Danny White said, who was a rookie in 1976. "We were old school guys that were being paid what we thought was a ton of money to play football, and they would let us come over and workout for free. We were going to have our own private workout facility and not charge us a penny."

When Ward arrived after he accepted the job, there were not a lot of guys hanging around the weight room. The first guy he met was safety Charlie Waters, who caught Ward's eye for the number of scars all over his body and his cerebral interest in total game preparation.

"He looked like Zorro had used his superior fencing skills on Charlie," Ward remembers.

Another player who was there that afternoon when Ditka was giving Ward the 50-cent tour was a balding, physically fit 6-foot, 188-pound white guy.

"Bob," Ditka said, "this is our safety, Cliff Harris."

The previous season, Cliff Harris had been named to his first NFL All-Pro team and earned his second consecutive invitation to the NFC Pro Bowl team as a safety. He was from Fayetteville, Arkansas, a graduate from tiny Ouachita Baptist, and he embodied the type of player who only the Dallas Cowboys seemed to be able to find. He was smart, cerebral, yet his style suggested he was a fearless opponent. His nickname was "Captain Crash," earned for his penchant to hit, and usually take down, whatever was in his way. Former Washington Redskins head coach George Allen called Harris a "rolling block of butcher knives."

Harris had one question for Dr. Ward: "How do you think you are going to make me better?"

This was exactly the type of scenario that former UCLA track coach Tom Tellez thought he was not built for and Ward was. Ward had coached established, high-performance Olympic athletes before, and at 43, he wasn't a kid who would be easily intimidated. But a pro athlete making money and aware of his own celebrity is not a college kid or an Olympian who performs in a more obscure sport.

"Well," Ward answered with his slight signature smile and quick shrug, "we'll find out."

• • • •

One of the first orders of business for Bob Ward after he arrived to the Dallas Cowboys was simply to not screw it up.

"The single biggest difference between college football and professional football is the intensity of the strength training," said Cowboys fullback Timmy Newsome, who played for the Cowboys from 1980 – 1988. "In college, you have to do other things other than play football. When you get to the NFL, it is all about the game, and most of it is training and preparation."

The Cowboys were a team that had won at least 10 games in seven of the previous eight seasons, qualified for the playoffs in nine out of 10 seasons, and won one of three trips to the Super Bowl. By this point, the Dallas Cowboys were America's Team. The conditioning coach was not the missing piece. This was a roster comprised of well-established veteran names from Roger Staubach to Drew Pearson to Charlie Waters to Lee Roy Jordan and Mel Renfro. Some of the NFL's most celebrated names from the '70s were on this team when Ward arrived. This was a group that knew how to be a pro football team, and at this point, along with Pittsburgh Steelers head coach Chuck Noll, Tom Landry was the single most respected man in professional football.

"Tom Landry was the innovator and he knew everything that we were doing," said the team's secondary coach, Gene Stallings.

Unbeknownst to just about everyone at the time, including Ward, was that this was an elite staff. Stallings later went on to become the head coach of the St. Louis Cardinals and University of Alabama, where he won a national title in 1992. Mike Ditka would eventually leave to become the head coach of the Chicago Bears, where he won Super Bowl XX. Offensive coordinator Dan Reeves would also leave in the '80s to coach the Denver Broncos, and he would eventually coach the New York Giants and Atlanta

Falcons. Assistant coach Dick Nolan had already been the head coach of the San Francisco 49ers and would eventually become the head coach of the New Orleans Saints before he returned to Dallas as an assistant.

Stallings played under Paul "Bear" Bryant at Texas A&M and was named the Aggies' head coach when he was 29. He came to the Cowboys in 1972 and, by the time Ward arrived, was well schooled in what working for Tom Landry was like.

"Coach Landry would watch every single practice reel of every single position – offensive line, defensive line, quarterbacks, wide receivers, defensive backs – and he would be able to critique everything we were doing," Stallings said. "He would just make the rounds. And, most of the time, we were right in what we did."

Landry had this way of being able to cut without a knife.

"We would go into a team meeting after a win, and by the time you left that meeting, I swear to God you didn't know if we had won or lost the game," Hall of Fame defensive tackle Randy White said of Landry. "We would watch game film, and Coach Landry would say, 'This position right here needs to do this.' That's my position. I'm thinking, 'Coach, I've been here for 10 years and you don't use my name?' Am I not going to play on Sunday? Am I going to get cut? He had this way of constantly keeping you on your toes and motivating you."

The one person on this staff Landry did not critique was Bob Ward, but he had a clear idea of what he wanted in terms of fitness from his players. Ward had not been with the Cowboys for too long when he came across a letter written by Tom Landry after the 1975 season:

A WORD FROM COACH TOM LANDRY

The only way, and I repeat, the only way to be sure that you will be able to take full advantage of this tremendous opportunity you have in professional football is to be in top condition … you must increase your strength and you must work at it now, between now and July 1st. Every week that slips by can never be recaptured as far as strength building is concerned. After June 15th wind endurance, muscular endurance, agility drills, etc., take priority.

It is my greatest belief that the greatest enemy a professional football player faces is FAT. Fat slows every movement of your body; it encases your muscles and acts as a brake when your muscles contract for action and movement. If you are underweight, don't make the mistake of trying to add size by adding fat. Such added fat is not muscle and cannot become muscle. Fat cells once added can never be removed. An athlete can reduce the size of fat cells but once added you can never lose the fat cell. That is why it is easier to get fat the second time around.

To lose fat so as not to weaken you, you must start now. To reduce in July and August is too late and will affect your performance. As an athlete grows older he automatically loses muscle mass, and even though his body weight is the same, he is carrying more fat and less muscle each year, which affects his performance. Example: In 1966 if you weighed and played at 250 lbs. and had approximately 10 lbs. of excess fat, in 1973 the same athlete weighing the same weight of 250 lbs. will be carrying approximately 20 lbs. of excess fat and 10 lbs. less muscle mass.

The Dallas Cowboys have been one of the best conditioned teams in the NFL; however, this year we are going to be the best conditioned team in the league. It will be hard to ask our players to give more this year than they have in the past. They have lifted weights; they have run cross country; they have been in top condition…and to ask them to give more this year than in the past is not easy; but unfortunately life is that way. Each year it gets harder and harder to win, and we must give more and more – both coaches and players.

All of the teams in professional football are gathering and following similar plans and trying to follow our method (our off-season conditioning program), but no team will work harder, with more dedication than the Dallas Cowboys.

Two additional thoughts I would like to leave with you…no matter how big, how fast or how strong you are, you will never give a consistent performance unless you are in superior condition. Excellent physical condition is the most important factor in competitive sports.

It takes approximately 13 weeks of general conditioning to prepare you for specific conditioning.

The time is now.

"The guy we had before Bob in that job – a guy named Alvin Roy – was good," Cowboys linebacker Thomas "Hollywood" Henderson said. "But then we got Einstein. Then we got Dr. Spock."

Not long after Ward accepted the position, he pored through the files, folders, and workouts left by his predecessor, Alvin Roy. Like most strength or conditioning coaches in the NFL at that time, Roy's philosophies of training were rooted in the basic fundamentals of working out – work, work, work, lift, lift, lift, run, run, run. As far as nutrition, it was just about that simple as well.

"Alvin believed in work, work, work. And, as soon as you finished, you did more work," Charlie Waters said.

"In training camp, we would go to breakfast, and it was steak," Cowboys wide receiver Butch Johnson said. "At lunch, you'd have steak. At dinner, you'd eat steak."

After one practice session at the Cowboys' former training camp facility in Thousand Oaks, California, Johnson was walking off the field with head coach Tom Landry.

"Coach, can I ask you something?"

"What's up, Butch," Landry answered.

"Can we eat something other than just steak?" Johnson asked.

"Butch, why would we change if it's been working?" was all Landry said.

That phrase could pretty much be applied across the board about damn near everything when it came to the NFL during that time. When Ward came to the Cowboys, it was still a time when weight training applied to the traditionally "bigger" players – the linemen, the linebackers; the other players may have lifted weights, but not nearly to the level they do today.

"I know that when I came into the NFL [in 1970], the wide receivers really fought against lifting weights," Cliff Harris said. "They really did not want to do it. The tight ends, the line guys – they were the weight lifters. The receivers didn't want to do it because they didn't like it and because they thought that by lifting weights they were going to add muscle, make them bigger, and slow them down. Bob was a big believer in weight programs designed around [free] weights."

That remains a common misperception of weight training even to this day. When Ward came in, that misperception had only slightly begun to change. Slightly. Ward's presence was not designed to "change things that had been working," but to modernize an area that had not yet been brought to professional sports, specifically the National Football League.

Despite Landry's considerable knowledge of football and conditioning, he also knew enough to know he needed to leave Ward alone and allow him the freedom to implement the programs and conduct the research he wanted. Ward was not subjected to the same type of scrutiny, observations, and critiquing as the other members of the staff. "We never really did ask him what he was doing," vice president of personnel Gil Brandt said. "We let him do what he needed to do."

Ward was hired to implement his programs, concepts, and ideas for the 1976 Dallas Cowboys players. And the coaches.

"I had never done anything like he gave us," Ditka said. "I really wish I had known him when I was a player. He would have put another four years on my career."

In his "office" next to the weight room and practice fields, Ward looked over the outline that Alvin Roy had constructed, and then he went to work. It was not as if Roy's methods were poor; the Cowboys were one of the most successful teams in pro sports by that time. Roy in his time was considered one of the best, if not the best, at his job. But, like anything, there was a way to improve. All of the research and studies Ward had either conducted or read said the same thing – football is entirely about explosion and quick bursts – meaning the training should prepare a person for those activities.

Ward immediately went to work designing a program based on what he had done at Fullerton and with the Elite Throwers Program (Men and Women) for the United States Olympic Committee. What he wrote down on a piece of paper would eventually transform professional football, the Combine, the NFL draft, and even the workouts for the weekend warriors.

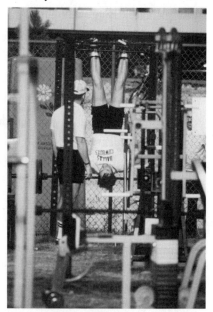

Bob Ward hangs upside down in a pair of anti-gravity boots as he instructs head coach Tom Landry on the benefits. Landry allowed Ward the freedom to implement the programs and conduct the research he wanted.

"When you see CrossFit today? That's what he gave us was - Beyond CrossFit," receiver Butch Johnson said. "All of that stuff – power cleans, box jumping, speed work – that is all CrossFit. We were doing that in 1976. He basically invented CrossFit before CrossFit was a thing. The only sad part is that he didn't patent it."

One of the first things Ward did with the Cowboys was to implement an increasing number of free weights. He added machine workouts – leg press, shoulder raises, and others had become popular by the mid-'70s. Bob was a believer in free weights for one specific reason: It focused on a person's total body strength, power, speed, core, and balance ... all of the things that today are routinely emphasized by professional sports trainers.

"Bob was definitely not old school, but when it came to free weights, he was very old school," Waters said.

In Ward's estimation, old school free weights were the best methods. Ward had purchased his own set of free weights – your basic dumbbell set from 20 to 150 lbs. – back in California and put them in Fullerton's "Weight Shed" that was used by students and other elite Olympic athletes at any time. When the Cowboys began their first training camp in Thousand Oaks, Ward simply had those weights re-located from Fullerton over to the Cowboys. They would remain with the team for more than a decade. Ward was applying plyometrics that had the Cowboys jumping on and off various box heights from 24" to 40" all designed to improve explosion training. These exercises have since been accepted as essential in starting, stopping, restarting, cutting, and faking – all key football moves.

"He changed the entire program when he came," Ditka said. "We were the most physically fit team in the league. We did things before anybody else did. The improvement in our guys was because of Bob, really. You say, 'Did everybody buy in?' They really did, and it was because of Bob. He said, 'I am going to help you,' and he did. I had never seen anything like what he was doing. Not at all. Not even close. He put years on a guy's career. And once other teams saw what we were doing, they all started to do it. It took a little while, but they all started to do it."

He was also an advocate for two amenities that were absolutely foreign to nearly every established coach in any sport at that time – rest and water. What are now universally accepted as essential for peak performance were then thought to be associated with laziness or quitters. Ward preached and put into practice a rest-work cycle that was still in its infancy in sports. Water, and more specifically water breaks, at that time was akin to using a piece of candy for a child; water was an incentive to do well or as instructed, not as something necessary to optimal performance.

One afternoon during a staff meeting, Tom Landry and his staff had a difference of opinion regarding their long held beliefs and what scientific research concluded. "Bob – water cuts into the time when we are trying to teach," Landry said.

"Coach, you do that and something happens and they will run you up the nearest yard arm," Ward said.

Back then, water was just water. Today, a water break is now called a hydration period, something no one skips.

• • • •

Joyce and their youngest daughter still lived in California, which allowed Ward to remain at the Cowboys facility for as many as 18 hours a day. He would stay there all day, every day, working out with the players. He weighed around 220 pounds, nearly all of it muscle. If he was going to sell something, he thought he'd better look like the results and believe in the products. Basically, a trainer worth anything can't be some fat, out of shape person. Ward was the picture of muscle strength. He was a gym rat who loved to work out and lift weights, and he knew this was the best way to connect with the players, to be on their level as far as what he was asking them to do.

As more and more players came around and met their new conditioning coach, he had them almost all confused. He did not yell. He did not bark. He

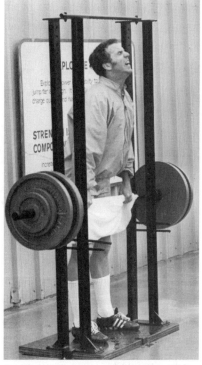

Dallas Cowboys Hall of Fame quarterback Roger Staubach performing heavy rack work in 1976 at a time when not all NFL quarterbacks were lifting weights.

was not going to tell anybody what to do. He worked out with them.

If he saw them using weight straps as grips around the bar he would say: "You consistently live up to the low standards you set for yourself."

Ward then would grab the bar and do it himself.

He approached Roger Staubach and simply asked, "Here – do you want to try this?" This was at a time when not all quarterbacks were lifting weights. Though Roger did express trepidation about some of the things Ward wanted, before long, he was doing cleans and jerks with the offensive and defensive linemen.

• • • •

One afternoon early in 1976 training camp, he approached safety Charlie Waters.

"Charlie, I am really worried about your speed," Ward said.

By that time, Charlie Waters was well established as one of the best safeties in the NFL. He had been in the NFL for six seasons, two of which he was a reliable starter. Waters was a good – not great – NFL player. By the time he met Ward, he was 28 and realized he was not going to be able to play forever. Charlie was raised in an underprivileged home in South Carolina by a pair of mostly uneducated parents, and he knew that football had given him everything. "I did not want anybody to take my job," he said. "I did not want to be a damn Wally Pipp."

In professional sports, to be "Pipped" is a verb synonymous with losing a job, mainly one in sports. Wally Pipp was the first baseman for the New York Yankees who on June 2, 1925, according to the legend, asked for a day off because he had a headache. The man who replaced him at first base was future New York Yankees icon, Lou Gehrig. Gehrig would start the next 2,130 games for the Yankees and not leave the lineup until May 2, 1939. His record stood until Cal Ripken broke it in 1995. No one in sports wants to be "Pipped."

"I knew I was not the fastest guy, and if Bob Ward could make me faster, I was going to do it," Waters said. "I knew I *had* to be faster."

Ward sat down with Waters and explained to him one of the reasons he could not run fast was that he did not envision himself being able to do so.

"Let's do it then," Waters said. "Let's go there."

Ward hooked up Waters to a giant piece of surgical tubing around his back and tied the other end to a goal post. It was a similar exercise he once used on Dave Murphy when the two were at Fullerton nearly a decade earlier. The tubing stretched like a guitar string, and Waters just kept backing up and backing up and backing up, to the point where he needed help. He made it about 40 yards and stopped. The tubing was tight, and Waters could feel the tension throughout his body.

"GO!" Ward yelled.

Waters took off running, and he could not even feel his feet hit the ground. Ward clocked Waters at 4.3 seconds – which in today's NFL is exceptional. He looked at Waters and said, "It's not how fast you go but how quickly you get there."

"I went almost face first into the goal post, but it worked," Waters said. "Not all of Bob's experiments went real smoothly, but most of them worked. He was so innovative and creative, and just different."

Waters continually practiced something Ward brought to the Cowboys – overspeed training – in 1976. That season, he was named to the NFC Pro Bowl. He would earn the same honors in 1977 and 1978. "I credit my emergence to becoming a Pro Bowler to Bob Ward," Waters said. "And he was the reason; I credit him for every bit of it. He brought a dynamic to me, and us as a team, that we had never experienced before in football."

Catching the attention of Charlie Waters was not especially tough. Waters wanted the help. But then there was the matter of impressing another player who no coach for the Cowboys could reach.

• • • •

Thomas "Hollywood" Henderson was born to be an athlete, an exceptional football player, and a giant pain in the ass for figures of authority.

"He was the single most impressive and unbelievable specimen I ever saw," said former Dallas Cowboys linebacker Bob Breunig, who played with Henderson in the late '70s. "He didn't need to lift weights. He didn't need to take steroids. He could do *anything* he wanted.

The team was lifting weights, specifically the bench press, outside the headquarters near the practice fields. The bench press rack was set at 350 pounds.

"Thomas ripped off however many in a row – it was unbelievable," Breunig said.

Henderson stood up and looked at some of his teammates who were in awe of his exhibition of strength.

"Guys, I don't need to do this," and he walked away.

"We were all watching and just like, 'Wow – that was awesome!'" Breunig said. "Some guys just have those genetics. I was good at lifting weights, and I could *never* do the things that Thomas did."

The guys that "have it" from birth, stereotypically, can be the most difficult people to coach or "reach."

"It can be done, but what I learned is that if you have a problem like that, it takes up about 70 percent of your time," the late Pro Football Hall of Fame San Francisco 49ers coach Bill Walsh said in an interview in 2005. "You have moments when you ask yourself, 'Why am I doing this?' You have to take it on with your eyes wide open and give yourself an exit strategy."

Walsh said he would take on such players when, he said, "I was young and impetuous and thought I could change people."

In 1976, Hollywood was a second-year player and the Cowboys had yet to ponder an exit strategy because they loved his ability. Players like Henderson are blessed with the ability from birth, take it for granted, and often times do not want to be told how to do anything. Hollywood Henderson had those all of those gifts. He was big, fast, and physical. He was one of those guys who could roll out of bed and be just as good in baseball, basketball, track and field, hockey, and auto racing as he was in football. He also was firmly aware of just how good he was.

He also had the gift, and curse, of getting in his own way. The 18th overall pick in the 1975 NFL Draft out of tiny Langston College, he was the type of off-the-grid player the Cowboys routinely found that other teams simply could not. He was the portrait of the talented but troubled athlete. He rebelled against authority and routinely called – and calls – the Tom Landry regime "The Cartel."

Henderson had a long battle with cocaine and often fought with Landry and his staff. But the Cowboys dealt with him because he was just so talented, and so good. There was, however, one guy on the Cowboys coaching staff who Henderson could deal with, and liked: Bob Ward.

Ward had dealt with plenty of successful athletes before, but he had never tried to tell a pro how to do his job. Some of these young men can be full of themselves, of ego, and are often surrounded by a fleet of sycophantic enablers who make taking instruction sometimes an impossibility.

Knowing that, one day earlier in Ward's time with the Cowboys, assistant coach Gene Stallings tried to get that point across when he pulled Ward aside and said, "Bob – this is not college. These guys are professional athletes. You can't talk to them the way you might have talked to the guys in college. You can't just tell them what to do."

It's worth noting that strength and conditioning coaches normally have an easier time establishing a relationship with a player than other members of the coaching staff because the position of a strength and conditioning coach is inherently on the side of any player, whether that person is a starter or a reserve. The only time this relationship may struggle is if the player prefers to workout and train on his own or use a system employing methods that differ from the team-appointed coach.

In 1976, players working out on their own or with their own trainer and their own "system" was an anomaly; it just didn't happen. Nowadays, most pro athletes have "their own guy" they work out with separate from the team coach. When Ward was hired, players at that point were not as sophisticated when it came to training and were far more likely to follow the strength coach on the team.

For some reason known only to a higher power, Bob Ward could reach Henderson without coming across as a bully, a dictator, or someone who was out to tell him he was doing it all wrong.

At that time in the NFL, players were not obligated to workout in the offseason. Many of them did, while many of them carried with them the intense fear of losing their jobs. Henderson knew better.

On the wall at the team facility was a giant chart listing every player's name, and every day he worked out there, they placed a large "X" by it. When Henderson arrived to training camp, there was not a single X next to his name.

"Call me a conscious objector," he said. "You had the guy trying to make the team with 50 Xs next to his name. Or the marginal player with 60 Xs next to his name. From a business standpoint, nowhere in my contract did it say I had to be there to workout."

Henderson loathed authority and disliked coaches, yet he did not perceive Coach Ward to be a threat. That itself was a major accomplishment.

"I gravitated to him because, unlike the other coaches, he did not treat you like a fourth grader at school," Henderson said, who to this day remains critical of everyone in Landry's regime but Ward. "You are scared of the teacher. You are scared of the janitor. You are scared of the head of the cafeteria. You were not scared of Bob. Bob would look at you and have something out there, a workout, and he would say, 'What do you think? Do you think this is something you may want to try?' It was not mandatory, but it was interesting. It was stuff I had never seen before. You *wanted* to try it."

Ward was just beginning to implement and flesh out the research and conduct studies on athletes and performance. The Cowboys let him do it, and there was no better lab than a professional football team with a stable of top tier professional athletes.

For a guy like Henderson, he set up a series of lights on the field for a routine 40-yard dash run. Most guys tire of this rather quickly, but Ward had it set up so guys would try to beat the lights as they lit up. Henderson was pushing himself not because a coach told him to do it, but rather to see if he could beat the lights. It was almost fun. Meanwhile, Ward was recording all of it. All the time.

He convinced Henderson to participate in the power clean exercises, among many others. Henderson knew he was a bad man, but also that Bob Ward could make him the baddest.

"I would go to training camp and after one week with Bob Ward I would be ready to whip everybody's ass; and then I'd see those guys who had 60 X's next to their name on the bus going back home [because they had been released by the team]," Henderson said.

As Ward would eventually learn, there was only so much he could do with a pro athlete versus the type of influence he could have on a college kid. Henderson, despite his talents and abilities, simply could not get out of his own way. He made the Pro Bowl in 1978, but was cut by the Cowboys after the 1979 season. His contemptuous attitude along with his drug use were too much for Tom Landry. Henderson played briefly in 1980 for the Houston Oilers and San Francisco 49ers but was forced to retire because of a broken neck.

"I will always be grateful for Bob Ward. He made me a powerful linebacker," Henderson said. "I had that fancy 'Hollywood' name, but I had power in that position because of Bob."

• • • •

Since Ward was not completely committed to the Dallas Cowboys beyond the two-year leave of absence Fullerton had permitted, subconsciously he needed to be impressed by the job.

Ward had been in sports for his entire life, either as a participant, or as a coach, or a scientist using state of the art computerized biomechanics. He had experienced every high and low that comes with an athletic game, so he was accustomed to the emotions attached to a sporting event.

There is, however, something decidedly different about an NFL game.

"Walking out of a tunnel and there are 70,000 people … and you are young and you are all jacked up," former Dallas Cowboys linebacker Bob Breunig said. "That is a big deal. It's a great time in your life. You are young. Your body is working. You are in great shape. It's the most unbelievable experience of your life."

The sounds, intensity, and emotions that are the part of an NFL game, which act like a drug to millions of people every Sunday in the fall, hooked Ward into thinking that a return to Fullerton was not going to happen. "The first time you come into a stadium as a part of an NFL team with 60,000 people. Are you kidding me?" he asked rhetorically. "There is nothing else like it."

There were periods, however, when this was not a given. Bob's arrival to the Cowboys was the equivalent of the kid going to kindergarten. Life and social transitions require time; his family support system not living with him in Dallas during that first year only compounded the problem. Ward suffered separation anxiety stemming from his childhood and the time spent away from his mother. Had Joyce not wanted to come to Dallas with their youngest daughter, he had made up his mind he would leave the Cowboys after the second year and return home.

He was lonely, which is why he spent so much time at the Cowboys' facility and in the weight room.

He was eventually befriended by the likes of Mike Ditka, Dan Reeves, Roger Staubach, and other players, but there was still a bit of a gap that first year. Most of the time, he was too busy to notice, but when there was down time, the isolation did affect him enough to ponder a return to California.

The team finished 11-3 in Ward's first season and won the NFC East. But they were upset at home in playoffs by the Los Angeles Rams, 14-12.

• • • •

In August of 1977, Ward's second year with the team, the Cowboys were playing the Miami Dolphins in a preseason game at Texas Stadium. Ward was standing around the 20-yard line – this was during a time when the NFL did not regulate who could stand on the sidelines the way they restrict those areas today. One of the reasons the NFL polices those areas so heavily now, other than because it can, is to reduce the possibility of injury when players run out of bounds.

During one play that preseason game, a Dolphins wide receiver was running toward the sidelines and the crowd of media photographers split, running to avoid being hit, though a collision was still inevitable. In most instances when there is a sideline collision between an oncoming player and a coach, a cheerleader, photographer, or official, the non-player always loses. It's usually graphic and can be painful to watch.

"The guy was coming right at me – I mean right at me – and I had to defend myself," Ward recalls. "So, I put my left forearm up directly in front of me to protect myself."

This is one of the few times the non-player won such a collision. Bob Ward was not your typical sideline observer. The man was built like a player.

"I didn't mean to do it, but it deflected him and knocked the guy down," he smiles. "The next week, we were watching the game film and all had a good laugh at that. But after that, I was no longer on the sidelines – they put me in the coaches' box to help the other coaches scout the opponent during the games."

After the second season, however, there was no way he was going back to Fullerton. The team won the Super Bowl with a 27-10 victory over the Denver Broncos, and Bob Ward had become an accepted part of the locker room fabric. That pull is nearly impossible to turn away from, and the Cowboys did not want Ward to go.

In the early part of 1978, the Cowboys participated in the now defunct *SuperTeams* event in Honolulu, Hawaii. This was a made-for-TV competition that had been created in 1973 by ABC; it had four teams, those who competed in the Super Bowl and Major League Baseball's World Series, face off in a sort of play-off to determine the overall winner. *SuperTeams* took place after the NFL's Pro Bowl. That year, the final round of competition pit the Dallas Cowboys, Super Bowl XII Champions, against the Kansas City

Royals, American League runners-up who participated in place of the New York Yankees, the 1977 World Series Champions.

Events included volleyball, running relay, tandem bike relay, obstacle course, swimming relay, war canoe race, and a tug-of-war. It was one of those events that would never happen today; the teams would never permit their under-contract players to participate in such a competition for fear of injury.

Because he wasn't a player, Ward was not invited, but the Cowboys players participating in the event paid for Ward to come. They called him their "secret weapon," but the truth is they liked him and wanted him to be a part of the fun. In a un-timed tug-of-war against the members of the Kansas City Royals that included Darrell Porter and George Brett, with broadcaster Keith Jackson saying, "We may be watching the ultimate isometric exercise." Ward was right along side players like Harvey Martin, Ralph Neely, Robert Newhouse, Charlie Waters, and Randy White.

The tug-of-war ended, called at 1 hour and 15 minutes.

"One of the reasons we wanted him to go was because we thought he could help with strategy; we were actually unsure of what to do," Waters said. "But he was engaged with us all the time, and he lived it all. I would go workout twice a day at the practice field, and there was not a single time he was not there. He never griped or complained about everything. It was like Pollyanna, but he was a weight guy, too."

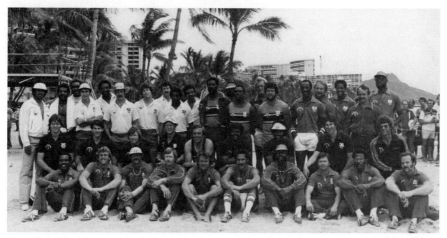

Bob Ward pictured with the "Super Teams" – players from the Kansas City Royals and Dallas Cowboys – in 1978 in Honolulu, Hawaii. Ward made the trip with the team; they called him their "secret weapon." The Cowboys and Royals ended up tying. Officials called the competition after a tug-of-war lasting 1 hour and 15 minutes.

As a side note – the Cowboys actually lost this overall competition against the Royals. The Cowboys lost because they lost in volleyball. When Ward returned to Dallas and the team's complex he was asked to report to Coach Tom Landry's office.

"Bob, you are from California," Landry said. "And you lost in beach volleyball?"

The players gave Ward a large oar from the competition as "Thanks," which he still has. Ward was not a player, but he had become a part of the Dallas Cowboys. He made the decision to end his tenure with Fullerton Community College and to relocate his family full-time to Dallas. He would remain with the team through 1989.

"For me to last 14 years in that job?" he muses. "I was blessed to work for Coach Landry and be a part of a wonderful coaching staff and players…I still can't believe that happened. There was not a position like the one I had in any professional sports team, not even today."

In a little more than a calendar year, the Cowboys had seen enough to know that Ward was doing more than simply earning his paycheck, he was doing something extraordinary for that position and for that team.

Ward's Words
Busting Ed "Too Tall" Jones

Of the many men I was honored to work with and next to with the Dallas Cowboys, no one meant any more to me than Jim Myers. He was the team's assistant head coach/offensive coordinator and offensive line coach. Like me, he was an officer in the Marine Corps; Jim served during World War II, was a strict military man, and a devout Christian who worked tirelessly for the Fellowship of Christian Athletes, the Tom Landry charity golf tournament, his church, and many others. I absolutely loved this man. He was a tremendous model for me. I was honored to speak at his memorial service when he passed away. Our houses were close by, and every day I drive by it, I give him the USMC salute for a job well done.

We were roommates together at those dorms during training camp in Thousand Oaks, California.

Jim was as loyal and as dedicated a man as I have ever met, and he was absolutely a no-nonsense guy. Coach Tom Landry was mostly stoic and unemotional; Landry was one of the guys who could really needle you without saying very much. He didn't need to because everybody knew he had absolute power. Jim Myers was like a USMC drill sergeant who was completely unafraid to get in your face. He was the opposite of Landry. Jim didn't cuss or swear, but he would let guys know if they were messing up.

At training camp, Jim was in charge of monitoring curfew – bed check. He loved doing it. If a guy returned to the dorms past midnight, they would get fined. The fine was normally about $500.

One night in the late '70s at training camp, where players did not always have cars, it was past midnight, and Jim was standing on the second floor of the balcony looking for guys to return. He sees this shadow, and it's a big shadow. It was Ed "Too Tall" Jones. Ed Jones stood 6-feet-8, and was the tallest player in the NFL. There was no way to miss that man, and his size made it impossible for him to effectively hide behind anything other than a truck.

Ed tried not to be detected; he would run and stop behind trees heading to the player's dorm, so we might not see him. He was Ed Too Tree Jones. Jim and I were both laughing at this until finally Jim, normally a screamer, simply said, "Ed – peek-a-boo. I see you, Ed."

CHAPTER **7**

APPLYING SCIENCE TO HIGH PERFORMANCE

*"The challenge is not just to build a company that can
endure; but to build one that is worthy of enduring."*
– Jim Collins

Not long after Bob Ward's first season with the Cowboys was over, head coach Tom Landry assembled his football coaching staff for a meeting. These meetings were quiet, and they followed a speak-when-spoken-to model that Landry had learned both in the Air Force and with the New York Giants. All of these men respected and revered Landry. And many of these men were of the generation that understood the chain of command and the necessity of keeping their mouths firmly shut until told otherwise.

Football is not war, but it is the sport usually most associated with combat. In team or group oriented combat, the person next to you is often the reason you will succeed, or the reason you die. Loyalty in this sense is paramount, and to a man like Tom Landry, it was something not to be ignored, or diminished. Landry stood at the head of the conference room and looked around at his staff. This was a serious room with serious men who were about the serious business of winning football games in the cutthroat world of the National Football League.

"I want to stress the importance of loyalty," Landry said. "It is important that everyone in this room is loyal to the organization, to each other, and to this football team. If we are going to be as successful as we want to be, we all have to remain loyal to the Dallas Cowboys. There cannot be anybody in this room who shows any disloyalty to this organization."

The room remained quiet, and individually, everybody wondered where Coach Landry was going with a message that, to them, did not require any reinforcement. This was not the first time Landry delivered a stern message to the staff. Landry held up a color picture so the entire room could see it clearly: It was a picture of sharply dressed Dallas Cowboys strength coach Dr. Bob Ward proudly holding up a pair of Los Angeles Rams underwear. Some friends in Southern California had taken the shot when he and his wife had recently visited and sent the photo as a gag to Tom Landry. The entire room cracked up giggling and laughing. Ward slightly blushed.

"Like I said," Landry said as he flashed a rare smile, "loyalty is the most important thing for this football team."

It had taken a year, but Ward had become a part of the team and a part of the staff. Likewise, the team became a part of him, and what happened to them mattered to him; he felt it when they lost. No loss bothered him any more than the Cowboys' upset home defeat to his daughter Shannon's favorite team – the Los Angeles Rams – in 1976. Between Roger Staubach and the "Doomsday Defense," this was a game they should *never* have lost. But Staubach threw three interceptions, and the Cowboys lost by two points. This was a reminder to Ward of what he learned decades ago playing ball – the difference between winning and losing is normally a decimal point of a fraction, and how people treat you.

The disappointment of the season-ending loss to the Rams was not even cold yet when Ward set out to write down what every single player needed

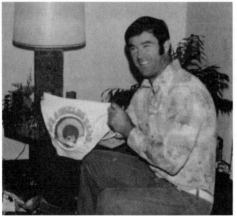

to do in the offseason. Normally, the standard operating procedure of a man in his position was to give every player a one-size fits-all workout, if that, and that was effectively the end of conditioning until the next training camp began. At that point in the evolution of football, teams were not uniform in giving a player an offseason workout program. Some teams did. Many did not. Some guys worked out. Many did not.

Bob Ward holding up a pair of Los Angeles Rams underwear – a gag gift given to him by friends. This photo would be used by Dallas Cowboys head coach Tom Landry to tease Ward at a staff meeting after Ward's first year with the team.

Absolutely none of that would happen in the current era of sports, on nearly any level. Today, every single professional athlete has a specific workout plan tailored to their specific needs. Personal trainers do the same for the 9-to-5 working mom or dad who wants to exercise at the local gym.

What the Cowboys found out was that Ward's program, rooted primarily in Eastern European and Russian methods, *worked*. What history would later reveal is the "Bob Ward Methodology" worked so well, everybody in the NFL would eventually copy what he was doing and it would still work more than 30 years later.

• • • •

Ward always felt if he was going to sell his program to players, he had to do it first to see if it worked. In that sense, he was Doctor Henry Jekyll – the infamous title character from the Robert Louis Stevenson classic book where the doctor took a potion he believed would succeed in exploring another side of a person. Ward never did turn into Jekyll's alter ego, the diabolical and murderous Mr. Hyde, but like Jekyll, he believed the only way to find out if something worked was to do it himself.

Ward worked out with every player on the team, including many Olympic athletes who came there to train, not only to demonstrate how to properly do a power clean or a jerk or a box jump, but to embody the benefits of the exercises. When he coached at Fullerton Community College, he built what was essentially a workout shed that was open 24 hours a day and operated on the honor system. Athletes at the school could work out there, as could pretty much any kid in the area who wanted to lift weights and train, and Ward worked out with those kids.

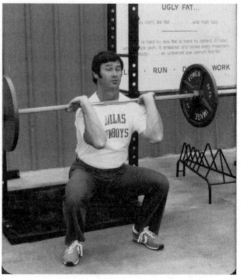

By the time he came to the Cowboys at 42, Bob Ward

Performing a front squat for players at the team's practice facility in Dallas in 1979, Bob Ward believed the only way to find out if something worked was to do it himself.

was the model of fitness and health. Early on during his tenure with the Cowboys, sporting long sideburns and black hair that covered most of his forehead, Ward conjured shades of actor Burt Reynolds in the 1974 movie *The Longest Yard*. At a minimum, Ward didn't look 42.

In 1974, he took his oldest daughter Shannon to the movies when they were still living in Southern California. Shannon was home during a break in college, and while in the theatre, she noticed a few friends from her high school days. After the movie, she began talking to one of the friends who asked, "Don't you think that guy is a little old for you?"

Shannon realized the friend had no clue the older man was.

"You think he's older?" she asked.

"Why are you going out with some 28-year-old guy?" he asked.

"That's my *dad*," she said.

Ward credits his appearance and health to nothing more than good genes and clean living since he was a kid. His biological father's horrible relationship with booze scared him away from alcohol. Despite the fact that Ward was raised in an era when the dangers of nicotine were unknown, his relationship with cigarettes was brief. He did smoke, but quit after only a short period in the early '60s.

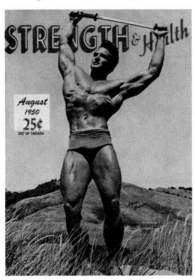

One of Bob Ward's first inspirations, 1950 Mr. Universe Steve Reeves. Ward had a copy of this magazine when he was a teenager.

Even into his 80s, the man appears to be in his 60s. Even into his 80s, he exercises every day, he doesn't eat junk, he takes vitamins. Even into his 80s, he still has definition in his biceps and calf muscles – all a result from years of lifting and exercise.

Ward figured if he was going to pass as an expert in his field, he had to look like the results he promised. Former USC All-American discus thrower Dave Murphy said of Ward, "The guy was an absolute stud."

From the time Bob was a teenager and bought a copy of *Strength and Health* magazine for twenty-five cents that featured on the cover 1950 Mr. Universe winner Steve Reeves, the man was a workout freak.

Not playing professional football did not prevent Ward from playing other sports after college. As his wife of over 50 years has noted – Bob is a total flop at sitting still. After he graduated from Whitworth College, Ward remained active in amateur sports, like martial arts, rugby, handball, weightlifting, and track and field for decades.

Long after his official amateur career was over, Ward was still throwing the shot. Still throwing the discus. Still throwing the javelin. Still clearing the bar on the pole vault. In 2002, in the 65 to 69 age bracket, he was the American record holder in the clean and jerk, the hammer throw, and five different categories of the weight throw.

He was *still* doing this after his 70th birthday – Ward would hold six world records in the weight and hammer throws for ages 70 to 74. In that time, he recorded world bests in the throws pentathlon and clean and jerk.

In 2002, he was named the "Field Athlete of the Year" by USA Track and Field for the age range of 65 to 69. And then when he turned 70, for the next four years he was named the USA Track and Field Athlete of the Year for the age bracket of 70 to 74.

At a minimum, the man always looked the part of the physically fit athlete.

• • • •

In his first season with the Cowboys, Bob Ward immediately did what Tom Landry hoped he would do – implement a program based on something far more sophisticated than a bench press or squat rack. Ward's views of football were rooted in what football is at its core – speed, burst, explosion. The only way to effectively prepare is to practice those three verbs. "Jimmy Johnson said it and he was absolutely right – 'do what you do best,'" Ward recounts. "If you are a pitcher, pitch. If you are a hitter – hit. If you are a golfer – golf. If you rush the passer – rush the passer. Do what you do and do it well; in other words, train with skill."

Even though the '70s was still the time of the Cold War, nearly everything Ward used was rooted in Russian and Eastern Bloc training ideals. Ward didn't know it when he was in college in the early '50s, but after World War II ended, the U.S.S.R. began to invest heavily in its sports programs. It researched and hand-picked young men to fill out its

Olympic rosters. When Communist Russia was still in the midst of a more romantic period rather than the cold paranoia that would eventually derail its government in the '80s, sports was fun. A man named Anatoli Tarasov began his career as the coach of the internationally famous Red Army hockey team in the '40s, and his training methods, while initially viewed as bizarre, eventually became widespread. By the early '70s, his team was the best in the world, and his training methods and coaching techniques were seen as revolutionary.

In 1974, a coach from America was visiting with him and asked him to reveal his coaching secrets. Tarasov looked at the man and said, "Do you think we have secrets? Today's secret is tomorrow's common knowledge. All you have to do is look. There is no secret in hockey. There is imagination, hard work, discipline, and dedication to achieving whatever the goal is. But there are no secrets, none at all."

Despite the lines drawn in the Cold War and the ostensible cut-off in communication between the West and the East, Ward said, "It got out. People talked. You can't help it."

Virtually everything Ward handed the Dallas Cowboys in 1976 was straight out of Mother Russia. In the 1982 edition of the *National Strength and Conditioning Journal*, Michael Yessis, who earned his PhD from USC, wrote a three-page study titled, "If the Soviets Had Football." Not that American football is an internationally widespread sport in 2015, but in 1982 virtually no one outside of the U.S. played the game. Yessis embraced and implemented Soviet training methods in the U.S. in a career that spanned more than 50 years; he worked with NFL teams such as the Los Angeles Rams, the Raiders, and the U.S. men's volleyball team. What he outlined in the article in 1982 is what Ward was essentially doing in 1976.

Bob Ward knew football is not war, but he approached football like a general planning for an invasion. "He brought this dynamic that we had never experienced in football," Cowboy safety Charlie Waters said. "It was the Eastern way of thinking of combat, of 1-on-1 fighting to football."

Ward likened his job to an army general planning for innumerable scenarios before an army took a beachhead. No one was dying, but the preparation for a football game could be carried out to far greater detail than it previously had been. When Ward's first season with the team ended, it was the first time he could sit down and draw up an individual workout for every single player on the team using computer technology.

Before the players walked out the door for the offseason of 1977, they each had to stop by to see Ward. Rather than visit or talk about what their plans were and provide advice about working out, he had drawn up a plan for everybody down to the coaching staff. *This* was new.

"When I was at Penn State, we didn't have any offseason workouts at all," said former Dallas Cowboys offensive lineman Tom Rafferty, who was drafted by the Cowboys in 1976 and retired after the 1989 season. "The first time I ever had an offseason workout, or something written for me, was from Bob."

As a result of the research Ward had conducted, he believed that not only did every player need his own individual workout to address that person's particular needs, but these workouts also had to be specifically tailored for the position.

Ward had drawn up charts and a list for the needs and demands of every position on a football team. "I had never seen anything like that," Cowboys wide receiver Butch Johnson said. "I had seen workouts before, but I had never seen anything that said, 'A wide receiver does this, so he must do this and this and this.' That blew me away."

In hindsight, it is rather obvious what Ward was doing. The needs of an offensive lineman *should* be different than those of a wide receiver, or a kicker, or a quarterback.

When linebacker Bob Breunig stopped to see Ward, he was handed a large stack of computer paper that was filled with data, numbers, and "the plan" – "This is what you need," Ward said. "And this is what we're going to do."

A computer printout, something that was itself still new, was not foreign to Breunig, but this "assignment" complete with detailed analytics was certainly uncommon. "It was a breakdown of everything you did that season; everything that Bob could measure and had been measuring all season long, it was all right there," Breunig said.

The second part of the computer printout was a highly detailed plan to prepare for training camp.

By this point the Cowboys were well-versed in Ward's theory that football was an explosion sport that necessitated workouts anchored around bursts, most notably jumps, acceleration, and sprints. Ward's work detailed a specific 90-day plan leading up to the official preseason start to the Cowboys' season.

It featured aerobic workouts, anaerobic workouts, a three-lift maximum for a bench press, among other things. Everybody on the team was handed one of these, from quarterback Roger Staubach to the punter, who was actually future Pro Bowl starting quarterback, Danny White.

Whether or not the player did the workout and followed Ward's outlined plan was entirely up to the player. A player such as Thomas "Hollywood" Henderson was not going to do anything he didn't have to do, so he didn't. A guy like Breunig, and most others, did.

"I wanted that last little piece in the worst way," Breunig said. "I had good workout discipline, and with Bob, I know I worked out harder. I was so obsessed with it, and I wanted to be fully prepared. What did this give me? As much as anything, it gave me the confidence to avoid injuries, and more than anything else, it gave you the confidence that you were ready."

Ward always preached effectively using time when it came to workouts – that training for the sake of training was not only a waste, but also counterproductive. In outlining the needs for every player, "the plan" included a three-phase cycle of post-competitive, pre-season and season. In today's era this is all rather common but in 1976, this was a new Ferrari.

The root of every program is five steps, and really it could apply to anybody in any walk of life, not just to football players:

1. Where have I been?
2. Where do I want to be?
3. How can I get where I want to be?
4. Am I willing to pay the price to get there?
5. ACTION

There were a handful of facets Ward introduced to the Cowboys that no other team in the NFL had implemented at that point – explosive training, running, sprinting, negative resistance, and specificity for the position. There is virtually nothing Ward implemented then that is not used in some variation today. His advances and theories on running and conditioning were one of the reasons the Cowboys hired him. They needed lifting *and* running.

Before, when football players trained to run, they just jogged.

"Bob was ahead of the curve enough to realize if we spend enough of our time jogging, we are spending time on learning how to be slow," former Houston Astros strength and conditioning coach Dr. Gene Coleman said.

"Why would you jog to prepare when all you are doing is learning and training to run slow?" he asked. "Football is entirely about explosion."

If you are going to be fast, practice being fast. Football is a lot of things – violent, fast, quick, but its plays are not particularly drawn out. Not long after Ward came to the Cowboys, he and a fellow sports scientist measured all positions analytically during an actual game.

Analysis of a Football Game:

Factors	Time/Distance
Game Duration (gross)	3 hours +
Game Time	60 minutes
Plays per game	50 to 70 plays
Actual playing time (20%)	5 to 7 minutes
Passing % of total (52%)	2.6 to 3.6 minutes
Passing time/play	2.3 to 5 seconds
Running time % of total (48%)	2.4 to 3.4 minutes
Running time/play	2 to 5 seconds
Kickoffs (4/game)	45 yards
Punts (6/game)	40 yards

Based on these measurements, one of the first items Ward changed when he joined the team was to modify the way the team ran; this was the specifically why the Cowboys gave him the job. His predecessor, Alvin Roy, was not a running guy. Football players generally hate running for distance, and in that era, guys were required to meet certain minimum standards in endurance. Before he arrived, the standard was the same for everybody – run 1.5 miles under 12 minutes. After Bob was hired by the Cowboys, he changed up the standards according to each position. There was absolutely no reason why a big, husky linemen needed to demonstrate the same type of running endurance as a wide receiver or running back.

His running workouts revolved around two concepts that seem so obvious now:

1. Football is based on repeated acceleration to specific field positions that in many cases end in collision.
2. Our integrated and maintenance programs must train these elements as well as the stamina to repeat these bursts at 30-second intervals of recovery.

He used the word "interval"; today, "interval training" is used in nearly every sport at every level and is something amateur athletes use with great success for weight loss. The Cowboys, all of them, turned themselves into sprinters *and* distance runners *and* weight lifters. "That was the part that we had never done before," quarterback Roger Staubach said. "If you looked at us, the Cowboys, the Bob Ward-trained athlete is in much better shape today than ever before."

As far as the specific core, he implemented one sit-up exercise that left many players so sore the next day they would actually complain.

When Ward arrived to the Cowboys, this was right before the start of the Nautilus and machine-weight explosion that hit the U.S. He wasn't necessarily opposed to such equipment, and he would implement some of it, but when it came to lifting weights, Ward maintains there is absolutely nothing better than free weights.

When Kevin Callaway arrived to the Dallas Cowboys in 1983; he did so knowing full well he was a long shot to make the team. He was an offensive lineman and a rookie free agent, after all. He was with roughly 100 or so other players hoping to make one of the few roster spots available. On a dot-matrix printer, Ward handed Callaway an individualized workout that carried him through every repetition of every weight he needed to complete. "By the end of the seventh week, I had gained just phenomenal strength,"

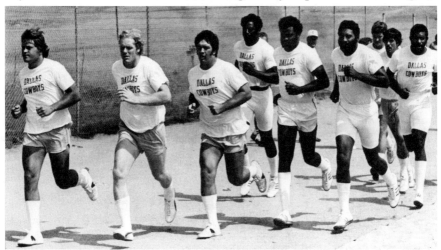

Thousand Oaks, California – The Dallas Cowboys doing the Coach Landry 1.5-mile run in under 12 minutes to determine the conditioning level of every player before the start of training camp. The standards changed once Bob Ward was hired.

Callaway said. "My seven weeks I spent with Bob Ward, that was the best shape I had ever been in my life. That was the strongest I had ever been in my entire life."

Regarding free weights, Ward believes there is nothing better than squats, dead lifts, bench press, and a set of barbells and dumbbells. He had guys jumping on elevated boxes of varying heights, something none of them had seen before. To work with these worked everything, up to and including the "core" – the concept is that it focuses on the stomach and the butt. "Core training," in the modern era, is a commonly used term and exercise.

"If you look at what guys like Bob Ward, and myself, and others were doing with squat racks and those things – that is what core training is, we just didn't call it that," former San Francisco 49ers and Chicago Bulls strength and conditioning coach Al Vermeil said. "There is nothing that strengthens a core like those exercises."

Ward stressed the players not use what are commonly called "weight straps" around the barbell. He wanted the players to have strong hands, and "weight straps" were a way to cheat to ensure the barbell doesn't slip from the grasp. "It was about tackling," safety Charlie Waters said. "He believed that if you could get a grip, you could make the tackle. He wanted your hands to be as strong as the rest of your body."

There was one particular game where Waters made a tackle simply by grabbing a player by his jersey and throwing him down. Ward threw up his hands and screamed, "There you go! It's the grip!"

What Ward put in that first offseason worked. In 1977, Ward's second year with the team, the Dallas Cowboys finished the regular season 12-2. In the postseason, they blew out their three opponents by an average of 21.3 points. They defeated the Denver Broncos 27-10 in Super Bowl XII.

"I know our offseason was the best in the NFL, and that had a lot to do with our regular season," Staubach said.

• • • •

A book called *Spine In Sports*, written by Robert G. Watkins, was published in 1996. Twelve pages in this book are dedicated to Ward's football workouts, nearly all of which he applied to the Cowboys. The study is titled "Trunk and Lower Extremity Strengthening For Football" by Robert Ward.

Ward writes:

> "... the most important protective element in playing football is not the strengthening of tissues but the way their collective strength is used. I have observed many elite football players over the years who overtrained the structural components (e.g., bench press plus 500, power clean plus 400) at the expense of nervous system control."

For instance, in the spring of 2001, Dallas Cowboys offensive guard Larry Allen benched pressed 700 pounds on one lift. It is a legendary one-time lift for a player who eventually would join the Pro Football Hall of Fame. "I was there with Larry that day, and it was special that it happened because we did it in a healthy manner," former Dallas Cowboys strength coach Joe Juraszek said.

Surrounded by his coaches and teammates, who were hooting, hollering, and encouraging him. It is fun to watch a man lift 700 pounds. But does lifting that much weight one time really do much for the football player? No. It just looks cool.

Ward writes:

> "Efficient use of the athlete's body movements would dramatically reduce the negative impact of improper handling of energy on the field, thereby reducing injuries and increasing performance.
>
> Many coaches waste valuable time and effort by spending too much time, especially during the preseason, on isolated factors (e.g., speed, strength, agility drills) and not enough on their integration into the game itself. Certainly, basic elements comprise the minimum skills required for a specific performance level. However, an increase in any one element does not guarantee a commensurate improvement in the skill."

When a researcher breaks down how little a football player actually does in a football game, it reinforces the notion that football is the most over-practiced sport in America. In 1985, one of Ward's Indiana University professors, sports scientist James "Doc" Counsilman, completed a study about the need for explosive power, which is something Ward specialized in and for which he is likely the most well-known. In a letter dated October 24, 1985, Counsilman wrote to Ward:

- "The football moves less than 20 minutes of a 60-minute game."
- "The average distance run by a backfield man is usually less than 15 yards. For example, the average gain per run by [Dallas Cowboys

running back] Tony Dorsett is about five yards, but he probably runs 15 yards to achieve a five-yard gain."

Some of these numbers have since changed. Specifically, the number of passing plays per game has increased as both college and NFL teams have adopted throwing as a primary means of moving the ball. The number of plays per game Ward cites in this study – between 50 to 70 – remains about the same in today's game. In 2014, the Philadelphia Eagles ran an NFL-leading 70.4 plays per game. The Tennessee Titans ranked last in the NFL in that category at 57.4.

The NFL remains rooted in trying to fit games in a three-hour block for television, meaning the number of plays will never vary too greatly from one decade to the next.

There is, however, one notable exception to the above study. Trumain Carroll played defensive end at Oklahoma State University from 2001 to 2005, and in 2015, he was hired as the head strength and conditioning coach at SMU. He was hired by SMU football coach Chad Morris for one specific reason – to train his football players to run more plays than ever before.

When Carroll played at Oklahoma State, he and his teams routinely had problems with one opponent – Texas Tech. Coached by Mike Leach, the Red Raiders were revolutionary in an offensive design that put a premium on tempo, speed, and the frequency of plays.

"I absolutely hated playing them," Carroll said. "In a normal game we would run 60 or 75 plays. Against Texas Tech, they would get you up to sometimes 100 plays. We had more guys cramping up in that game than they would all season. On the flight back after we played them, we would have guys in full body cramps on the plane.

"More and more teams are doing what they do and are running more plays than ever before. You see Baylor, Oregon, and other places running that offense that wants to snap the ball fast. The whole idea is you can snap the ball as fast as possible to pressure the defense. The guys who run that offense have to be in better shape to do it."

When Ward began to breakdown an NFL game by a fraction of a second with a fellow researcher named Dr. Ralph Mann, what they found is football is not what it appears to be. Mann was an Olympic hurdler who competed at the 1972 Summer Olympics in Munich, Germany. He later earned his PhD in Biomechanics from Washington State University. When he studied a completely broken down and dissected football game, he told Ward: "I thought football was a contact sport. There is not that much contact. It's more about avoidance of contact."

Time Duration By Functional Category	*Categories Applied to Football Event Time*
Impact	100 msec
Reaction/Force	100-300 msec
Quick Play	30 msec – to 2 seconds
Play Time (avg.)	2 to 10 seconds
Prolonged Play	10 to 60 seconds

How ironic. Football is equated and known as the most violent sport in North America. It is a game allegedly full of nothing but contact, yet when a play is broken down, the collisions are infrequent, but they can be both brutal and life altering.

The idea is to completely break down every single element of a player and what he does in a game to maximize preparation, training, and fatigue management. It is something that every trainer does today in their respective sport. But beyond just breaking down each act, or motion, of a football player – does his method to maximize a person for the game fly today?

In a section of his 1996 study, Ward discusses the "Seven Dimensions of Training":

1. **Centering**

   "*Centering* (the first dimension of seven dimensions discussed later) is a term used to describe a physical and mental dynamic that is in a constant state of flow. This concept has been expressed by many dissimilar groups in various disciplines or sports. It can be likened to the calm in the eye of the hurricane or the internal attention of the master performer in any skill."

This is not necessarily about core training, which is something that has become a main focal point for every professional and weekend athlete in today's era. "It's like a storm – the body is a tree and it's the center of gravity around which all of the limbs move. *That* is centering," Ward explains. "That can go from the concrete to the abstract. The abstract could be your thought process, but there could be a center point, which could move. I

ob Ward as a 5-year-old.
e was living with his
andmother at the time.

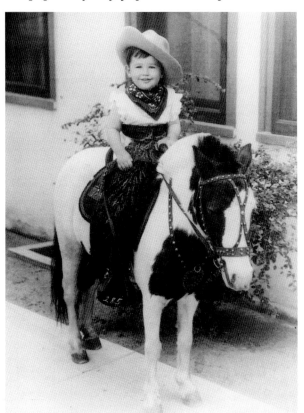

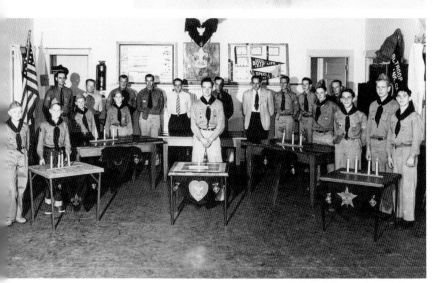

b Ward's Boy Scout troop in 1947 in Burbank, California. Ward figures his involvement
the Cub Scouts, Boy Scouts, and a local church provided him with a role model to follow:
hat's who my fathers were — the 'Scouts."

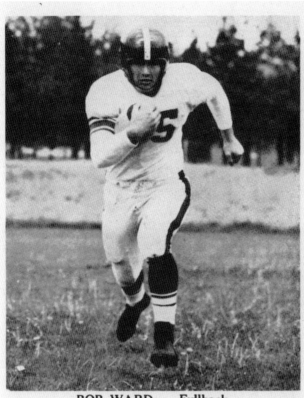

Fullback Bob Ward pictured in a Whitworth College game program. Ward also played linebacker on defense.

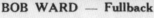

BOB WARD — Fullback

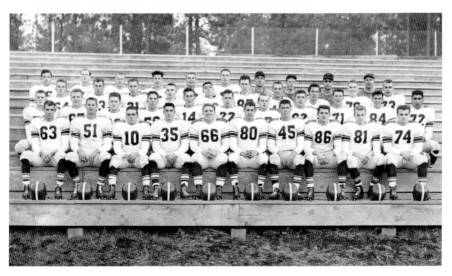

The 1954 undefeated Whitworth College football team. Ward was one of two Whitworth players named to the initial NAIA All-American football team. He was selected as a running back.

Bob Ward pole-vaulting at Whitworth College. Ward would eventually go on to coach track and field at Fullerton Community College, which opened the door to his future with the Dallas Cowboys.

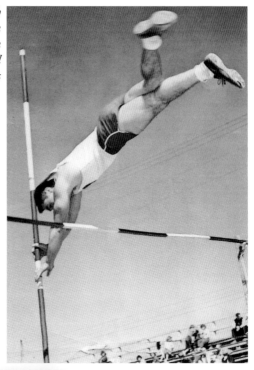

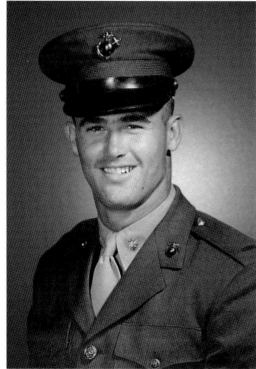

The Korean conflict ended shortly after Bob Ward was drafted in 1953, but Ward would remain in the active service until 1957. He trained in Quantico, Virginia – where he also played for the Marines' base football team and ran track.

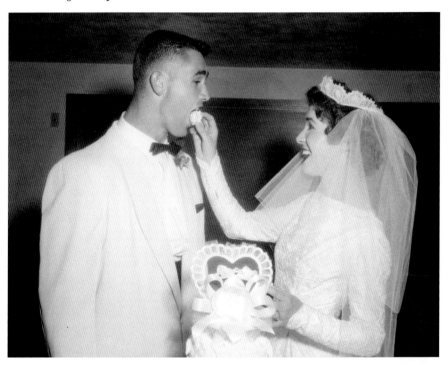

The Wards on their wedding day – June 16, 1956.

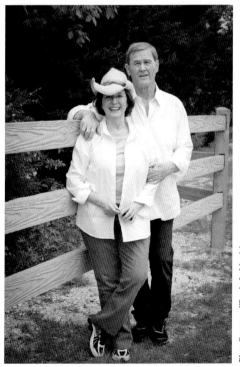

Bob and Joyce Ward – the two have been married nearly 60 years.

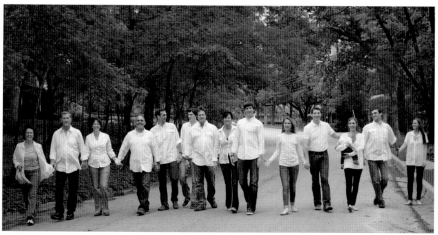

The entire Ward family, four generations.

Photo Courtesy of Teruko LaMendola

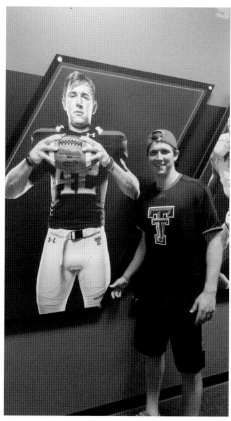

Taylor Symmank, Bob Ward's grandson, a punter-kicker at Texas Tech University, though he didn't learn to punt until he was in college. Before his senior year at Texas Tech, Taylor was named the Big 12 preseason punter of the year.

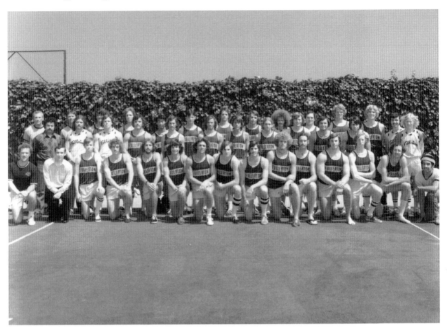

The 1974 track and field team at Fullerton Community College, coached by Bob Ward with assistant coaches Tom Gilmer and Al Feola. The team won the California State Track and Field Championship.

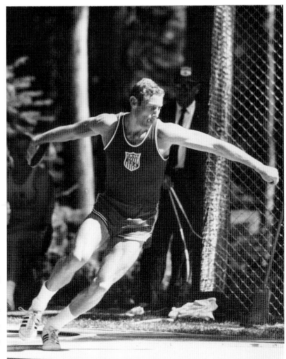

U.S. Olympic decathlete Rick Sloan here throwing the discus. Ward coached him at Fullerton Community College. Sloan would eventually become the track coach at Washington State.

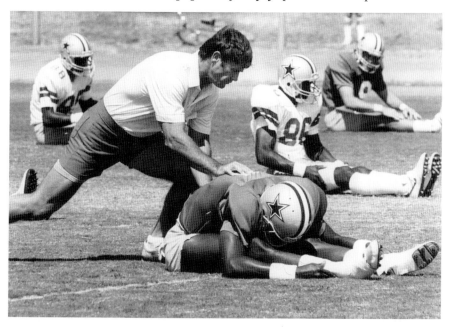

Bob Ward warming up a Dallas Cowboys player before practice at training camp in Thousand Oaks, California, in the late '70s.

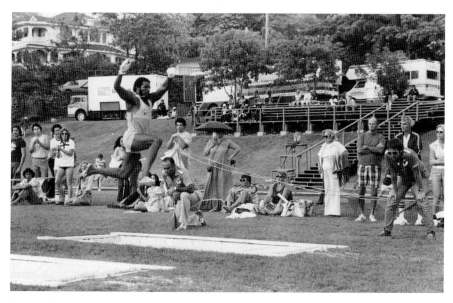

Dallas Cowboys linebacker Thomas "Hollywood" Henderson in the long jump at the Super Teams competition in 1977.

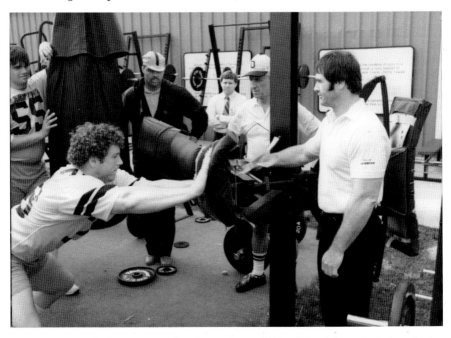

Bob Ward and the "reaction machine" next to good friend Jim Myers (wearing the hat to Bob's immediate right). Ward would later attach an accelerometer to test how hard a player could hit the pads.

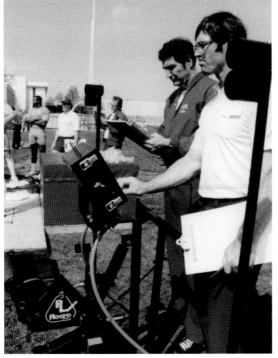

Cowboys assistant coach Gene Stallings standing with Bob Ward at practice in Dallas in the late '70s. Stallings would go on to become the head coach of the St. Louis/Phoenix Cardinals and win a national title at the University of Alabama.

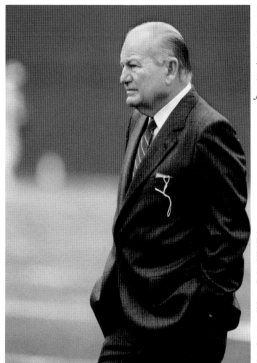

Tex Schramm, president and general manager of the Dallas Cowboys from 1960 until 1989. Schramm hired Tom Landry and Gil Brandt. Together, the three guided the Cowboys through their first 29 – largely successful – seasons.

Photo Courtesy of Manny Rubio/USA Today

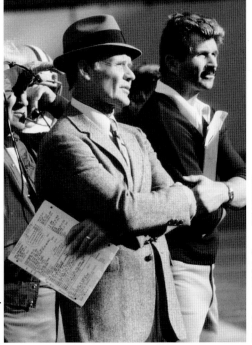

Dallas Cowboys head coach Tom Landry (left) with assistant coach Mike Ditka (right) on the sideline during the game against the Pittsburg Steelers in October 1979. Ditka would later become the head coach of the Chicago Bears as well as the New Orleans Saints.

Photo Courtesy of Malcolm Emmons/USA TODAY

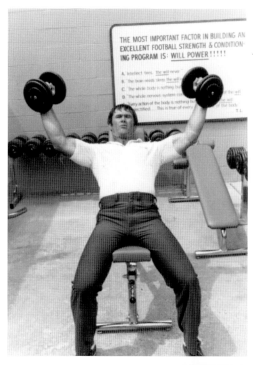

Bob Ward performing incline flies with dumbbells at the Cowboys' practice facility in Dallas.

Bob Ward filming a Cowboys quarterback during a practice in training camp in the late '70s. Ward recorded as much as he could, whenever he could. The more data he had, the better he could help each individual Cowboy improve for his particular position.

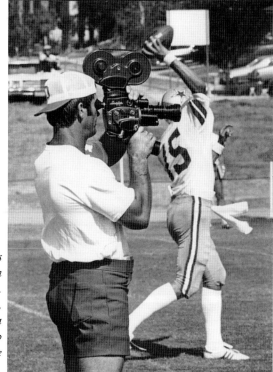

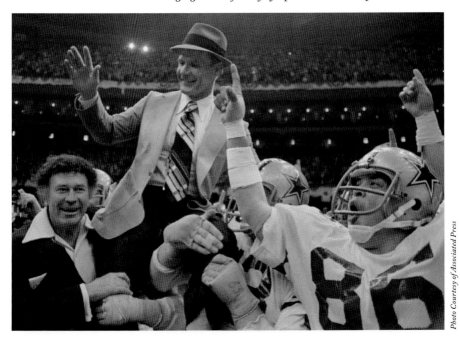

Photo Courtesy of Associated Press

January 15, 1978 – After the Dallas Cowboys defeated the Denver Broncos 27-10 in Super Bowl XII, Dallas head coach Tom Landry rides on the shoulders of his players in celebration.

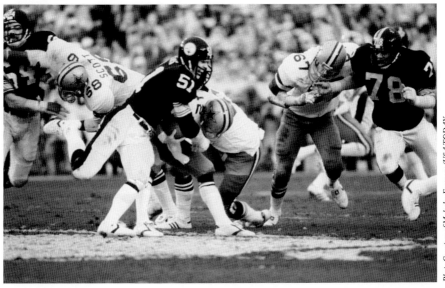

Photo Courtesy of Malcolm Emmons/USA TODAY

Super Bowl XIII – January 21, 1979, Pittsburgh Steelers linebacker Loren Toews (51) tackling Dallas Cowboys quarterback Roger Staubach (12). The Cowboys ended up losing the game 35-31. During this time, the Steelers linemen were known for their bulging biceps; the team is widely considered a pioneer of steroid use in the NFL during the '70s.

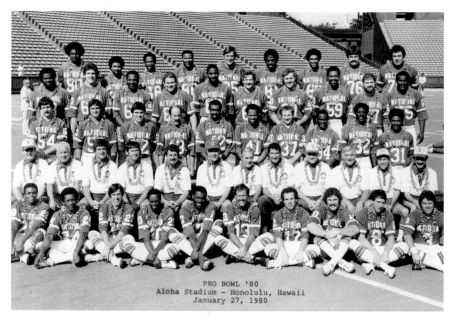

PRO BOWL '80
Aloha Stadium - Honolulu, Hawaii
January 27, 1980

Bob Ward accompanied the Dallas Cowboys staff to coach the 1980 NFC Pro Bowl team in Honolulu, Hawaii.

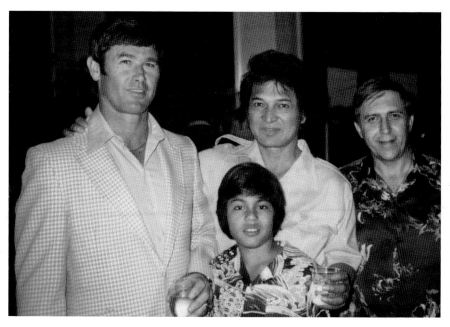

At the 1980 Pro Bowl in Hawaii, Bob Ward pictured here with legendary Hawaiian singer Don Ho (middle) along with Dallas Cowboys trainer Don Cochran (right). The younger man is Don Ho's son.

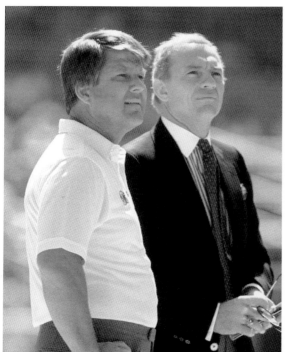

Bob Ward was one of the few coaches Jimmy Johnson (left) retained on his staff after Jerry Jones (right) bought the Dallas Cowboys in February 1989.

Photo Courtesy of RVR Photos/USA TODAY

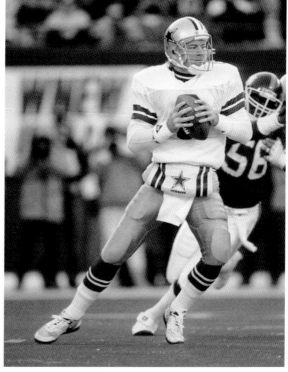

December 16, 1989 – Dallas Cowboys quarterback Troy Aikman against the New York Giants. The game where the Cowboys could not advance the ball 36 inches for a touchdown.

Photo Courtesy of RVR Photos/USA TODAY

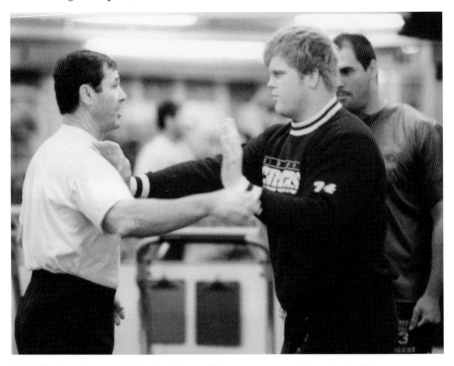

Bob Ward working with the San Diego Chargers as a consultant in the '90s.

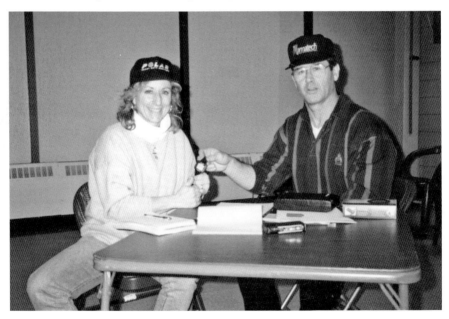

Bob Ward with Dee Dee Jonrowe, noted three-time Iditarod competitor – and to-date holder of the fastest time recorded for a woman, in Willow, Alaska. This picture was taken when Ward was conducting research for Mannatech in the late '90s.

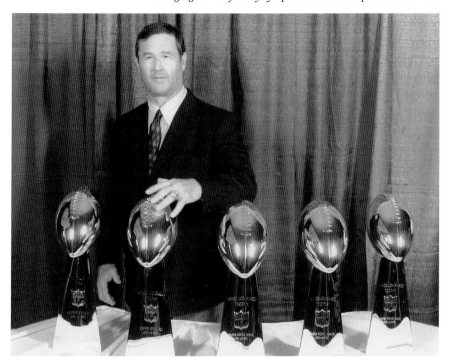

The Dallas Cowboys' five Super Bowl trophies, with Bob Ward touching the 1977 trophy the Cowboys won while he was on staff.

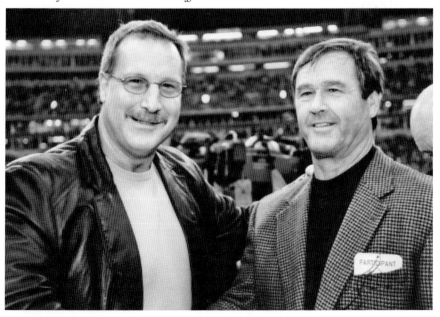

Dallas Cowboys Hall of Fame defensive tackle Randy White with Bob Ward at a Cowboys reunion event in the early 2000s.

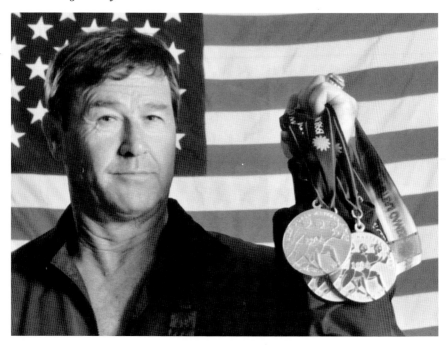

Holding up his medals after winning three golds at the Nike World Games in Eugene, Oregon in 1998. Bob Ward won awards for hammer throw, shot put, and weight pentathlon for ages 65 to 69.

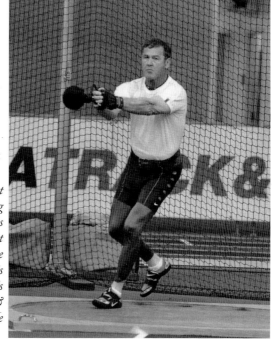

Bob Ward has made fitness part of his life from a very young age and it shows. Here he is competing in the 20 lbs. weight throw in the early 2000s, one of the five events in the Masters Throws Pentathlon. Ward holds six American Masters Track & Field Records for the 75-79 age group.

know this concept is right. This is based on the fundamental that the tissue gets stronger. You work the entire body in balance."

Ward is a believer in centering not only when it comes to training but also in life. Former Dallas Cowboys safety Cliff Harris, who worked with Ward in the late '70s and remains a controversial non-inclusion to the Pro Football Hall of Fame, mentions one thing instantly: "It's hard to describe this but having a center balance," Harris said. "That is the one thing Bob emphasized was a focus on balance all of the time. It was not only about weight balance distribution to be in a more balanced position to make a tackle but to have balance in life."

2. Specificity

"There is a tendency to view specificity as a modern concept. However, if a thorough historical study were conducted, it would reveal that human beings have used it from the beginning of time. For example, if drum skills are the desired outcome, it takes only common sense to practice on the drums, not the violin. An understanding of the principles of music certainly helps, but there is no substitute for hands-on practice time with the instrument to develop the neuromuscular processes involved. That the literature reveals many advocates of this principle is a given. The question, however, is how to apply it in the training program. Again, the answer is simple: practice the skill, and the necessary training benefits will develop accordingly."

Ostensibly what Ward is saying is if you want to be good at tennis, you primarily play tennis. That is specific sport and muscle training. But in this section, "specificity" requires further explanation because the word is counter to what a decreasing number of coaches stress today – play everything rather than one thing. Today, it is not totally uncommon for little league athletes, sometimes starting at the age of 8, to pick one sport and commit to that year round.

Little league baseball coaches will often coerce their players to commit – sometimes with contracts – to play just baseball and nothing else. Basketball and now even football are often the same way. It has killed the multi-sport or seasonal athlete beginning before middle school.

Ward is not advocating single-sport athletes from the time the kid is seven. The single sport specialization, in 2015, is often blamed for the anecdotal increase in burnout among younger athletes, and statistical proof of severe injuries as well. In 2014, there was such a dramatic increase of elbow injuries to pitchers in Major League Baseball that the American Sports Medicine Institute felt the need to issue a press release. The number of ulnar collateral ligament reconstruction surgeries – normally called "Tommy John" – was so dramatic that renowned sports surgeon Dr. James Andrews went on a press tour speaking out against what on the surface sounds like "specificity." The crux of the argument is that year round pitchers are pitching too much, too hard.

"We studied fatigue in youth baseball, and we found out that if a kid played with fatigue he had a 360,000 percent increased chance of injuring his throwing arm," Andrews said in an interview in August of 2015 in Dallas. "That can be in any sport. It's event fatigue, meaning too many pitches in a game. Seasonal fatigue, too many innings in a season. Year-round fatigue, meaning too many games. The risk factors relate to specialization and professionalization of youth sports."

Andrews "credits" the success of professional golfer Tiger Woods for the growing number of parents who have made their child's athletic career a priority from a young age. "How many Tiger Woods are there?" Andrews asked. "He's one in a million."

To have such vast global success at a young age, Tiger was the poster of the phenom teen with the guiding parent. He spawned countless hopefuls who soon realized there is but one Tiger.

Andrews has his own clinic dedicated to surgery on athletes in Alabama. He said he has seen a steady rise in adult-like injuries to youth athletes, more than ever before, which he blames on the increase of the specialization in youth sports. He said it is not uncommon for parents to ask for a serious and invasive Tommy John procedure on their teenage son in the misguided hopes that it will make the kid's arm stronger and more attractive to college baseball or pro baseball teams.

Andrews has also seen a rise in torn ACLs (anterior cruciate ligament in the knee) among young girls that are playing year-round volleyball, soccer, and basketball. He has also seen a rise in burnout as he believes more teens are quitting sports because they are simply sick of playing.

"I want to keep youths in sports. Being operated on as a young kid is a big, big step back," Andrews said. "I have been working on this for years, and I am not sure I have made a dent in it. We have to keep putting pressure to cut this back. What you don't want are for the lawyers to take over. Major League Baseball is involved, and that carries a big, big stick.

"Some sports do require early specialization - gymnastics, maybe tennis, maybe swimming. Look at [PGA golfer] Jordan Spieth – his parents would not let him specialize in golf until he was in college. They made him play multiple sports; he had to be an athlete first."

Ward's category of "specificity" is not anchored on doing just one thing. Ward is a big believer in too much of a "good thing." He is of the generation that played multiple sports and remains a believer in that philosophy. "When I was growing up you had seasonal sports and offseasons," he said. "But a football coach wants the guy to go out for track. Or wrestling. It's not identical, but they are working the fundamental movements of the body that enable you to improve the A, B, and Cs of your fundamental body movement, including the basic energy system's capacity."

There is only one Bo Jackson or Deion Sanders – the two most successful multi-sport athletes in the past 30 years. This should not preclude others from trying other sports.

For instance, deceased Baseball Hall of Famer Tony Gwynn, who was a career .338 hitter for the San Diego Padres in 20 seasons in Major League Baseball, often credited his success as a hitter to strong wrists that he acquired playing basketball. Gwynn was an All-Conference player for the San Diego State Aztecs basketball team in the early '80s.

Dallas Cowboys Pro Bowl quarterback Tony Romo was actually a better basketball player in high school than he was a football player. In his senior year at Burlington High School in Burlington, Wisconsin, he was named his conference's player of the year – ahead of Caron Butler. Butler, who played at Connecticut, would later become the 10th overall pick in the 2002 NBA Draft and play 13 NBA seasons. Romo was not offered any basketball scholarships and, instead, accepted a partial scholarship to play football at Eastern Illinois University.

"You do the skill," Ward explains, "but the smart one fills in where there are weaknesses. You do the skill, but you do not over do the activity. You get that by working on everything. By playing all different kinds."

In the 2015 NFL Draft, 256 players were selected. According to

University of Iowa assistant football coach Seth Wallace, 244 of those players were multi-sport athletes in high school.

"The hard part is to know when you draw the line on doing too much of the same thing, or too much of other things," Ward says. "You only know that by doing it."

When the Dallas Cowboys relocated their team offices and headquarters from central Dallas to the suburb of Valley Ranch in 1985, Ward was the one who designed the workout and training areas. Included in that were a pair of handball/racquetball courts. He also had tennis courts and a basketball court installed as well as a boxing ring. He *wanted* people to play different sports.

"We would play handball and turn the heat up to 120 degrees," Cliff Harris said. "We used it for eye-hand coordination and for conditioning."

3. **Efficiency**

"The law of efficiency is a natural effect of applying the first two dimensions. It guarantees the athlete the most efficient use of training time. The training effects produced will have the greatest direct impact on the skill or sport. Because precise stresses are being placed on all the body's systems, the effects will be efficiently developed. Consequently the tissues required for the task are being strengthened in the exact patterns of usefulness."

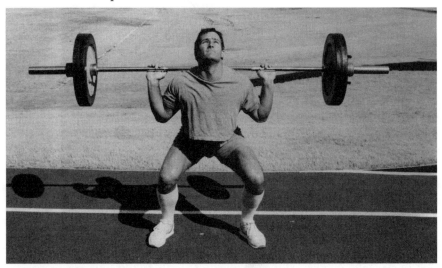

Dallas Cowboys safety Bill Bates performing a back squat at the track facility designed by Bob Ward at the Cowboys' new facility at Valley Ranch in 1986.

Research had not evolved to the point where fatigue, exhaustion, and rest were considered. Ward simply believed if you can achieve the same result in 30 minutes as opposed to 90 minutes, choose the former.

4. Planes and Tensions

"Most exercise programs do not stress the horizontal plane that runs parallel to the ground, and few exercises include a twisting motion around the vertical axis... Alternating dumbbell exercises designed to produce these motions provides excellent training."

When Ward wrote this study, he felt that exercises were still rooted in the basics of the vertical. Bicep curls go up and down. Squats are up and down. Jumping jacks, pull-ups. Ward believed in right/left, side-to-side motion. He believed in twisting. Today, it would be virtually impossible to find a workout program for any professional or amateur athlete that does not include or stress these principles.

5. Balance Focus

"My opinion is that a natural body wisdom produces the anatomic changes best suited for the skill. However, a fine line exists between this ideal and a condition that would create an imbalance or undesirable adaptation in the body."

If this sounds redundant to No. 1 it is only slightly. This portion is more geared to specific exercises. It does, however, re-emphasize balanced muscle expansion and growth.

Basically, figure out what your body can do and build around your frame and not somebody else's. Listen to *your* body.

6. Exercise Selection

Nothing Ward writes here would ever be rejected by a modern day strength and conditioning coach. He is a believer in four basic elements around which to build any program for any person.

"1. Exercises that improve strength and power of muscles, ligaments, and bones

2. Exercises that improve anaerobic and aerobic capacity

3. Exercises that increase range of motion

4. Exercises that improve neuromuscular functioning, agility, balance, and coordination"

This is neither complicated, nor is it terribly sophisticated.

7. Program Development

The following is about as rough as Ward ever gets; he writes in this section:

> "For various reasons, too many programs have failed to coordinate all the essential training resources into a comprehensive program. Thus this model may expedite a solution to this problem in programming. In addition, further studies may reveal that much of our so-called scientific training regimens are unnecessarily fragmented and/or redundant and therefore have little value except for adding variety to our programs."

Ward then writes a detailed list of what such a program should include: Basic Training, Functional strength/power training, Ballistics training, Plyometrics training, Sport-loaded training, Sport speed/quickness/speed endurance, and Overspeed training.

Would something that was published in 1996 fly with a professional or Division I college football team in 2015? SMU strength and conditioning coach Trumain Carroll read it and concluded it would. Although there are some minor adjustments and advances that have been made since its publication, Carroll concluded that Ward's premise and solutions are still valid today.

"It's about explosion. It's about the lower body. This would work," Carroll said. "Really, since this was published, it's not that much different."

For Carroll, the differences today compared to 1996 come down to the individual trainer, the coach, and their philosophies toward eating and relaxing. "You still do have those guys that are training for numbers rather than what is best for the athlete," he said. "There are still trainers out there and strength coaches that just want to be able to tell their head coach, 'This is what my guy lifted or this is what our guys are squatting' when it has no real benefit to the guy.

"The truth is, today it's not that much different than when he wrote this. The only real difference is the toys that come with it."

• • • •

There was an additional facet to the "Bob Ward Methodology" that remains decidedly Bob Ward. The man was unafraid to try anything outside of the weight room. If a player thinks something can work, even if it's just one player, then it works.

"Bob would try *everything* under the sun," said former Dallas Cowboys offensive lineman Brian Baldinger, who played for the team throughout the '80s. "He was a bit out there in that regard. He just really didn't want to be put in a box and told to train a guy in a certain way."

Something Ward went out of his way to do was extend his program out of the weight room. *Way* out of the weight room, over to the Far East, to the circus, to a yoga studio, and in one case, to the existential. In an effort to constantly stimulate and draw the Cowboys players back to the practice facility in the offseason, he came up and introduced a wide range of programs that had nothing to do with a squat or sprint. Or football for that matter.

"Football can be monotonous and boring, like any other job," former Cowboys fullback Timmy Newsome said. "That's what made Bob so good at his job. He constantly varied it up and looked for ways to keep you interested. It's funny – I never heard a single player complain about the things he was doing. Some of things he was doing really did re-energize guys. It made you focus on things that are important. You need new wrinkles, and Bob was spectacular at that."

A knife may not be allowed in an NFL game, but the practice of throwing one could be beneficial. Or Bob thought it had the potential to be beneficial. By the early '80s, martial arts training was already a part of how the Cowboys were teaching players. Ward had a boxing ring installed at the team's practice facility and was teaching Thai Boxing. Then, Bob decided to add throwing knives to the routine.

One afternoon, he had one of his favorite and willing lab rats – Randy White –work with an expert in the field of throwing knives. It was about this time that some of the members of the Dallas Cowboys coaching staff looked at Ward like he was an idiot … again.

"Why are these guys throwing knives at a board?" assistant coach Gene Stallings asked after one practice where Ward has players lined up to throw Chinese knives. "What does that have to do with football? I have absolutely no idea what throwing a knife does to help a football player."

Ward picked a spot to set up the target on the practice field in Dallas. He placed it directly in front of the corrugated fence that fans would routinely watch through or above. Randy White threw one knife, and it went right through the fence. "I could see my job going away and me going to jail," Ward said. "I still don't know what I was thinking doing that." There were fans leaning over to watch him throw the knives he was throwing in their direction.

So knife throwing remained on the Bob Ward platter of athletic training, but he picked a different spot. Ward added stick fighting to the training regiment, too, to improve total body coordination.

"The hardest part Bob had with some of these things was breaking down the mental barriers we had about it because we had never seen it," defensive tackle Randy White said. "Once you got past that, then you could really see how they could help you."

Most of these unusual football activities went fine until one afternoon when the padded stick fighting between Randy White and Thomas "Hollywood" Henderson grew so fierce the two got into a fight in the locker room. White was mad that Henderson was beating him, but despite Henderson's many God-given physical skills, there was a reason White was nicknamed "The Manster." White picked up Henderson and literally shoved him in his locker stall.

Among some of the other "out there" ideas Ward introduced to the Cowboys was a professional skate boarder, a yoga instructor, a juggler, and a reaction-timing device. Some worked better than others.

The juggler was a bomb. "That one didn't work too well," Ward said. The idea of a juggler was to work on eye-hand coordination.

As is so often the case in big-time sports, people "want in." It is completely common to find an extra agent, a publicist, a psychologist, a life coach, a free throw coach, or any specific coach or whoever insisting that if they are part of the franchise, they can help the team win or make their organization better. When it came to the professional juggler, he wanted to be with the Cowboys. So he kept bugging and pestering head coach Tom Landry until the head coach flatly told Ward, "Bob – get this guy off my back."

When Ward introduced yoga to the Cowboys in the late '70s and early '80s, the exercise was still mostly an obscure series of Indian-rooted stretching and posing. Today, it's a massive cash-cow industry with benefits reaching beyond the physical to the mental and spiritual.

Not long after Ward arrived, he had players sit in front of a computer screen for one particular peculiar drill they had never seen before. This was in the mid-'70s, a time when computers were not omnipresent. A player would sit down in front of the screen; they would hold paddles in each hand

and have sensors just beneath both feet. When a flash would appear on the screen, they would react with the appropriate foot or hand displayed.

Rookie backup quarterback Danny White set the team record by doing it all, successfully, in 30 seconds.

"Danny – have you ever played a musical instrument?" Ward asked him.

White looked at Ward like he was an alien and said, "As a matter of fact I took eight years of piano lessons as a kid – what does that have to do with football?"

"You play piano and your brain tells your mind what to do and when that happens you tell your hands and feet what to do quicker," Ward said.

"OK – I agree with you," White said. "But what does that have to do with football?"

"It's simple – the faster your mind processes something, the quicker you can tell your body to do something and make a decision faster and better," Ward said. "It makes you a better decision maker."

White paused and thought, "This was absolutely 100 percent validating to my mom who made me take piano lessons when I was a kid. She would not let me quit when I really wanted to quit."

White is convinced that Ward is correct when it came to these mental, brain exercises.

"I was a better quarterback because I took those piano lessons," he said. "Maybe not for any other position in football but for a quarterback, it's all about decisions. And making them accurately and quickly. That may be more important than being an accurate passer. All of it takes a backseat to decision making. Every other position on the field knows what he is going

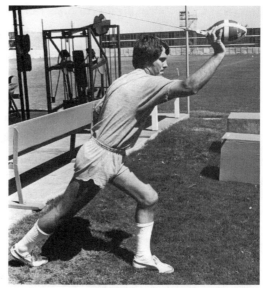

As it turns out, taking piano lessons as a kid actually helped groom Dallas Cowboys quarterback Danny White for the problem solving he would have to do as a quarterback. Here is White working on a drill to improve tissue strength of the throwing system in the late '70s.

to do before the play begins except the quarterback. Once the ball is snapped, the quarterback has to react to everything and make a decision based on everything else.

"I had never thought about any of this until I met Bob. Then, all of this made sense to me. It gave me confidence in Bob, and for a player to have confidence in their coach like that is everything."

Ward's method proved so successful that when the Dallas Cowboys built a new practice facility in 1984, team president Tex Schramm had Bob Ward fly back from the team's training camp in California to Dallas to talk. They were drawing up plans for the headquarters and offices; Schramm wanted Ward to design the weight area and the exercise portion of the facility. What Ward designed was something that so many teams would copy and emulate, including the team that fired him.

At the team's facility in Dallas suburb Valley Ranch, Ward had the Cowboys build a large track that encircled the back portion of the facility. The track included hills, dips and turns. There were several stations where the players would stop on the track to do pushups, run through tires, or other exercises that looked similar to boot-camp style military training. He had the team install a "sand pit" where players would sprint through sand, like running on a beach. The whole concept was designed around explosive training.

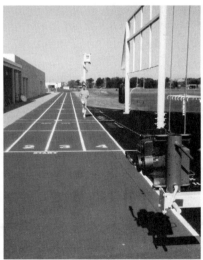

The track was one of many things Bob Ward designed and implemented at the Cowboys' practice facility in Valley Ranch, Texas, in the mid '80s. The team will be moving to a new facility in Frisco, Texas, in 2016.

• • • •

One of the most famous plays in the history of Major League Baseball began with a man visualizing it happening. In the 1988 World Series between the Los Angeles Dodgers and the heavily-favored Oakland Athletics, the A's led Game 1 4-3 in the bottom of the ninth inning. Pitching was the best relief pitcher in baseball, A's closer Dennis Eckersley.

Dodgers manager Tommy Lasorda pulled a desperate move and called on outfielder Kirk Gibson to come off the bench to pinch hit. Although Gibson had a sensational season, he had suffered a serious hamstring injury in the National League Championship series against the New York Mets and could not play in Game 1 of the World Series. Gibson watched the game from the Dodgers' clubhouse and was livid when he heard NBC sportscaster Vin Scully say he could not play. Gibson summoned a clubhouse guy, grabbed a bat, and went to an indoor cage to see if he could swing the bat. He could. Barely. He could not bend over to put the ball on a batting tee, but he could just barely swing.

He informed Lasorda he could hit. With two outs and a runner at first base, Lasorda called on Gibson. Before he walked out of the dugout to the on-deck circle, Gibson visualized himself hitting a home run. He visualized himself not feeling any of the pain that had reduced him to a bag of immobility.

"I told myself when I stepped out onto the field that the ovation and the environment would be outstanding and I wouldn't hurt anymore, and it was true," Gibson said in an interview with *ESPN.com* on the 25th anniversary of this famous night. "I knew when the opportunity came up; mentally, I thought I could do it. I just knew it. It was my calling. It was like someone was telling me, 'C'mon, let's go. It's time to do your thing.' I believed in it."

Gibson forced Eckersley to a 3-2 count, meaning if he threw a ball he would at least draw a base on balls. On the next pitch, Gibson took a swing and launched a ball over the right field wall for a game-winning home run and one of the most famous plays in Major League Baseball history. Gibson would not play again in the series, but the Dodgers would pull one of the biggest surprises in World Series history by defeating the A's, 4-1.

Most of this championship is credited to Gibson's shocking home run, which all began with his practice of visualization – a practice Ward believed in when he came to the Cowboys.

Visualization is not an easy practice; a player, or person, has to believe in it for it to actually work. Ward believes it can work for anybody. A few years into his tenure with the Cowboys, he offered something called a "sensory deprivation tank." It was just that – a giant tank of water that a player would rest in. It was a white fiberglass box – eight feet long, and four feet wide and four feet high. One at a time, for about an hour, players would enter what linebacker D.D. Lewis called "The Think Tank."

The Philadelphia Eagles had installed a similar tank, which cost about $3,500, one year before the Cowboys did in 1981. The Cowboys took it a bit further. They had a hole cut in the top of their tank and put a TV there.

"I know it sounds strange, but you would float there in salt water," safety Charlie Waters said. "It was quiet. There was soft playing music. And then he would put on videos of you making good plays or the stuff you needed to learn for the game. You would float there in this really calm atmosphere, and you would watch yourself doing your job really well."

It was akin to floating in space. The ears are under water, which allows a person to hear themselves breathe, which helps with relaxation. Tom Landry tried it, and even though it was eons away from his coaching origins with Vince Lombardi, when the two were assistants, he said, "You just have to have an edge someplace."

This does not mean everyone signed off on this across the board. One of the creators of a California-based company that researched visual stimulation was highly critical of Ward and his implementation of this practice with the Cowboys. In an article to *The New York Times* in 1981, Steve DeVore said what Ward was doing was "a gimmick" and that what the Cowboys were doing was "not scientific at all."

Ward had met with the company before installing it with the Cowboys. What he was implementing was not a direct copy of DeVore's plan; basically, DeVore was upset that the Cowboys had not paid him money.

Despite the concerns expressed by a handful of researchers and graduate students about Ward using these tanks, nothing ever came of it. To read about it, it creates the visual of the horrible psychological torture scene from the disturbing Stanley Kubrick movie *A Clockwork Orange* where a jailed hoodlum has his eyes pried open and is subjected to a long series of violent images to deter him from criminal behavior.

Objectors to this sensory-tank practice thought this was some form of mind control exercised by the Cowboys. "Dallas feels they have an infallible organization; except for one thing – the players. If they could play without the players, they could win every game," former Dallas Cowboys defensive end Pat Toomay said in an interview with *The New York Times* in 1981. He played for the Cowboys from 1970 to 1974, and for three more teams from 1975 to 1979.

In practice, the sensory deprivation tank was just one more device to help a player improve. Ward was not sure if it would work on everybody, but if it helped one, then it would be worth it. "Supposedly this helps concentrate on maximizing learning. It helps reinforce good behavior – the good parts of what you do in a game," he said back then. "Good shot. Good throw. Good pass. The mind really doesn't know the difference between the physical and the mental ... supposedly."

It was mostly about relaxing, clearing the mind. Visualization has become a rather standard practice in sports today, but it does not mean it affects everybody with the same rate of success as, say, Kirk Gibson and his famous home run. The power of positive reinforcement and believing good things will happen, however, is something that Ward stressed then and now.

• • • •

Of all the facets he introduced to the Cowboys, there was one that was so far off-the-grid, or above-the-grid, it may have been too much for football and its coaches and its players. In 1976, in Dallas, Ward met a man named Walter Covert who, while a student at the University of Alabama, delivered drinks to football coach Paul "Bear" Bryant. Ward struck up a relationship with Covert, who calls himself "The Number Coach."

At the time Covert met Ward, he was working with the long defunct Dallas Tornado soccer team, which had an office in the same building as the Cowboys. Covert was the promotions director for a team that played from 1967 to 1981. There was also a Playboy Club in the same building.

Covert is really a numerologist, mathematician, and an environmentalist. He says he has worked with football players, basketball players, college teams, pro teams, Hollywood actors, businesses, corporate leaders, and marketing consultants. As to which ones? He would rather not say. He said he has worked with government programs. As to which ones? He would rather not say.

He believes in numbers and that life can be explained through astrology and numerology. Covert believes a tarot card can explain the numbers on the back of a player's baseball, football, basketball, or hockey jersey. Numbers can be exchanged for letters, not to mention their mystical properties. It's not that much different than some of what former First Lady Nancy Reagan believed when she was in the White House with the late President, Ronald Reagan.

When Ward met Covert, the latter was in his 20s. His personality was a non-stop vortex of energy, ideas, and concepts that go way beyond the traditional thought process in sports, business, or damn near anything on this earth. Ward was receptive to Covert. What Covert believes and preaches is decidedly *not* for everybody. For example, Covert thought Ward was psychic, a visionary.

"Bob is a Cancer, and a Cancer is by far the most intuitive thinker there is," Covert said.

Covert introduced to Ward a handful of healing modalities from pulsating electromagnetism, oxygen therapies, clean water, and yoga breathing, to radionics. In turn, Ward introduced some of this to the Cowboys. Not everybody was sold on Covert as a Cowboys consultant. In the early '80s, when Covert would be seen with Ward at the Cowboys offices, grizzled and crusty linebackers coach Jerry Tubbs would say, "There's Bob's guru."

• • • •

The "Bob Ward Methodology" that strength trainers use today is rooted mostly in Cold War Eastern European training, and like those researchers and scientists, it goes far outside of conventional thought. It pushed and pushed and pushed to include anything that might work for an edge. For that reason, many of those once novel practices have now become standard order in 21st century sports.

Ward's Words
The Best Players

During my career, I worked with Olympic athletes and pro football players, and the best pure athlete talent I ever coached was Herschel Walker. He was the very best, and he was a do-it-your selfer. Psychologists classify it as "heuristic" – enabling players to learn on their own. Coaches should learn that learning is a do-it-yourself project. He was one of the guys I seldom, if ever, tried to train or coach. I did offer my conditioning suggestions. Herschel was just an exceptional athlete, and an example of self-directed, self-motivation. He was so good I didn't have to do anything. I just watched and encouraged him. He was a receptive guy, but he was a Lone Ranger. I didn't touch him much; I didn't have to. I wonder how much better he would have been had he not had a couple of injuries at the University of Georgia.

I had him from 1986 to 1989, and everything you have heard or read about that guy was true. He said he could 1,000 sit-ups, 1,000 pull-ups, and 1,000 push-ups a day. I never saw him do it, but I have no doubt that he could. Herschel Walker was one of the first guys to do things like ballet. He made everything look so easy.

There are too many to list and count, but here are some of my favorite weight room work out partners.

1. *Randy White, defensive tackle.* Start with him. He was the best. He worked so hard, he would try anything, and he was so open-minded. That was one thing that made him so good – he would really listen, and he constantly wanted to be better. He once went 15 three-minute rounds with a Thai boxing expert I brought in – that would test the spirit of any high performance athlete.

2. *Charlie Waters, strong safety.* Charlie was probably the smartest; he was intellectual and practical. He was so savvy, and he worked so hard. He would do and try anything you wanted him to do and more. He was an artist – he painted, and he was a thinker. He was a wonderful player to coach and work with; he was like a sculptor – he fashioned himself into an All-Pro player late in his career.

3. *Mel Renfro, cornerback.* By the time I got to the Cowboys, Mel's career was almost over. But he was just an amazing, naturally God-gifted athlete. We had similar backgrounds, he was a track star as well as a great football player at the University of Oregon. I loved working with him. He could really do it all – run, lift, and jump. You would think because he was an old-timer he might not be receptive to some of the things I was teaching, he really was. He was a wonderful player to coach.

4. *Roger Staubach, quarterback.* Based on off field tests only he had good scores for a quarterback, not at the top of the curve. When the game started, however, he was like a man who ripped off a car door to save a car accident victim. On game days, Roger was the Wizard of Oz. He understood better than anyone I ever worked with what he had to do. He was such a great influence.

   He was a good company man, and an ex military guy. He had hurt his shoulder before I got to the Cowboys, but that didn't really hurt him as a player. He just had natural gifts for playing quarterback. If you analyzed his talents, like at a combine, he wasn't at the top of the curve. He wasn't the fastest or the best at the jump, but he had the quickness, the mental capacity, and the ability to motivate people. Not many have that. He was one who optimally used his resources, a guy who never skimped on training and preparation.

5. *Todd Christensen, fullback. Most people forget he was with the Cowboys; he was a second round draft pick out of BYU in 1978, but he got hurt in the final preseason game of that year. We worked out together that season, and he really was a special athlete. He was a very smart guy; he was big, fast, tall, and he had fantastic hands. He was in the wrong position. The Cowboys wanted to convert him to tight end, but he didn't want to because we had Billy Joe Dupree, so we released him. The irony is he eventually went to the Oakland Raiders where he became a five-time Pro Bowler as, you guessed it, a tight end.*

6. *Drew Pearson, receiver. I have to put him on this list because he was one of those guys who constantly surprised you with what he could do. He was not the biggest or the fastest or the strongest, but Drew was one of those guys that could simply do it. He was not like any guy I really ever worked with before or since. I wasn't with the Cowboys in 1975, but whenever I watched Drew make the NFL's most famous "Hail Mary" catch to beat the Minnesota Vikings in the '75 playoff game I always think, "That's Drew." Drew was one of those guys who just figured out a way to make the play. He had a lot of the "measureables" – he was fast, he could jump – but he had this intangible to be able to make the catch.*

7. *Bill Bates, safety. A conditioning coach's dream. Bill did everything I asked him to do and more. He went the extra mile on and off the field – note: Bill took the most explosive hit I have ever seen on a football field and survived.*

8. *Bob Breunig, middle linebacker. Bob and I were born the same day, the 4th of July, albeit 20 years apart. It was a relationship made in heaven that has lasted from 1976 to date. Working with Bob was an educational experience. He was and is a perfectionist. Bob's preparation and application to football was evident in the Cowboy's "Doomsday Defense"; these skills ultimately led him to become All-Pro. Bob's work ethic carried him into a very successful career in commercial real estate..."Breunig Commercial."*

9. *Cliff Harris, free safety. Cliff was one of the first players I met in 1976 at the Cowboy practice field on Forest Lane. When Mike Ditka introduced him to me as their new conditioning coach, his first words were, "How do you think you are going to make me better?" A shaky start that developed into a great relationship. Cliff was a man who knew how to play, and he was a formidable tackler. He was respectfully called "Captain Crash." He knew what he needed to do to train and prepare, but he was willing to take what I suggested to add to his All-Pro talents. It was a pleasure to work with Cliff.*

CHAPTER **8**

THE ANALYTIC APOSTLE

"The goal is to turn data into information,
and information into insight."
– Carly Fiorina, Former CEO of Hewlett Packard

Jackie Smith was itching to leave for the day after Dr. Bob Ward had put the veteran tight end through a series of tests to measure everything from body fat to explosiveness. Jackie Smith had been an NFL Pro Bowler five times and had already played 14 seasons in the NFL, all for the St. Louis Cardinals. He was 38. He had come to the Dallas Cowboys for this his final NFL season and what he felt was his one shot at a Super Bowl. At this point in his career, why he was doing any testing at all was beyond him.

Here was this conditioning coach, running all of these tests to tell him he was aging, slowing, and not explosive. Ward printed out an enormous stack of computer readouts that included all sorts of charts, graphs, and numbers. Ward handed him the dot-matrix computer printouts and Jackie Smith just shook his head.

"Bob I can't read any of this," Smith said. "Can't you just tell me whether I'm alive or dead and let it go at that?"

What Ward handed Smith in 1978 looked eerily similar to homework. At that time, players were still mostly accustomed to reading a playbook, not doing math assignments. Ward had handed Smith a compilation based on "measurement techniques." At that point, "measurement techniques" had been around for many years, but guys like Jackie Smith and nearly every other player in any sport were either completely unfamiliar with them, or their exposure to them was minimal. Today, there is not a coach, a player, a general manager, or a fan who is unfamiliar with "measurement techniques." They just go by another name – analytics.

Measuring *any* game has existed since the origin of any competitive activity – it is more often called "keeping score." The measurement just evolved from tracking the score between teams to "keeping score," so to speak, on every player in every potential situation; today, technology quantifies sports and individual players by "measurement techniques." Few things in sports revolutionized games as much as quantifying something beyond the score.

• • • •

Of the contributions Ward made to the most popular game in North America, none was any bigger than applying "measurement techniques" to the players themselves on and off the field. After Ward arrived in 1976, he put computers to work to quantify all of the resources a player needed to play his selected position on the field, improve each player's performance, and to eliminate the many mistakes routinely made in evaluating the players by making the intangible resources tangible.

Ward was one of the forerunners in the information deluge in sports, all in an attempt to predict the future. What Ward was doing, which was called measurement and evaluation at the time, would not be called "analytics" for many years after his arrival, but analytics has helped transform both modern business practice outside of sports and the way we play and view sports today. It now encompasses all levels of every ball game, has created a contentious sports debate of "old school" versus "new school," and is responsible for a new sector of sports' industry.

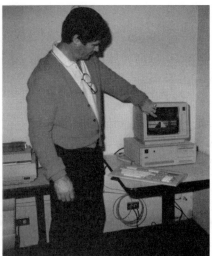

"There is absolutely no doubt he is the one that brought science to football," said Dr. James G. Disch, who also earned his PED from Indiana University in Biomechanics. At Indiana, his concentration was evaluation, statistics, and research. Disch eventually became a professor at Rice University in 1973 and would later join Ward in conducting studies and research on the Cowboys and U.S. Olympic Committee (USOC) Elite Throwers.

Bob Ward's computer, which was linked to other computers throughout the team's headquarters at Valley Ranch. Ward kept a wealth of data on each player in order to pinpoint specific areas for improvement.

"He is the founding father. He is the one that put the NFL on the track to sports science. It wasn't just a bunch of old jocks knocking heads. Everybody does it in different ways now, but he is the one that introduced players to modern science and then taught them how they could use it to get better at what they are doing."

• • • •

Ward's search for and learning the meaning of numbers began way before he went to the Cowboys.

"All sports have numbers and stats – all of them," he still believes. "It's a matter of finding them." When he was working on his Master's Degree at the University of Washington, his thesis was essentially a study in analytics. It was titled, "The Effects of Participation in Selected Physical Education Activities on the General, Athletic Ability of Male Students at the University of Washington, 1959."

He began his doctorate work at USC, under noted biomechanist Dr. John Cooper, and then followed Cooper to Indiana University to pursue his PED in Biomechanics and Measurement and Evaluation (another name for Performance Analytics).

He packed up his two daughters, his wife, and their Afghan Hound and moved from Southern California to Bloomington for one year and two summers to satisfy the university's requirement of one year of residence to finish his degree. It was in Bloomington where he started to research in a field of study that is now more commonly called "Sports Science." He had already earned his master's degree from the University of Washington in Physical Education, and he was certain there was more there than he was seeing or could even measure.

This field included scores of disciplines, and its origins actually trace to the time of the Civil War, when it was something called "anthropometric" studies. It took a more definitive shape in 1892 when Harvard University created the first exercise physiology laboratory in the U.S. It was at that time when researchers began to combine the measurement of the body, of strength and cardiac capabilities. The studies at Harvard then focused on oxygen metabolism as well as muscle structure and function – nothing as it related directly to winning a basketball game or kicking a field goal. At the time, baseball, football, basketball, hockey, and other sports were still mostly recreation activities, if they existed at all.

Measuring athletic ability began at the turn of the century; it is not a coincidence that all of this research and measurement was hastened considerably by the birth of the modern day Olympic games. On April 6, 1896 in Athens, Greece, the Olympics was brought back from its origins in ancient Greece to the world. A young French Baron named Pierre de Coubertin proposed that the Olympics return. The Olympic Games were created in ancient times as part of a religious festival every four years. The Olympic Games were stopped in 393 A.D. by Roman Emperor Theodosius I, because he wanted to defeat paganism. By the late 19th century, such concerns no longer seemed relevant, so at an international sport conference in Paris in 1894, de Coubertin pitched for a return of the Olympics. It was unanimously approved. The International Olympic Committee (IOC) was formed, and Athens was chosen as the birthplace of the modern Olympics. The Winter Olympics were added in 1924.

The modern Olympics changed sports forever. No longer was "playing ball" just for recreation; there was a new motivation to look for an edge and to strive to be the "best in the world."

• • • •

Exercise physiology was a field of study both nationally and abroad in the '60s when Ward was at Fullerton Community College. By that point, he had already been conducting extensive research on Olympic athletes in Southern California. Even though it was "just a junior college," Fullerton attracted internationally renowned track and field athletes such as Bill Neville, who held the NCAA record at Occidental College in the discus and, for a while during the '60s, ranked third on the all-time world list; U.S. Olympic weight lifter Russ Knipp; NCAA All-American shot putter, Dave Murphy; and Tom Hirtz, who would become a two-time weight lifting champion.

When he was at grad school at Indiana, Ward and his brother Paul conducted a study titled "An Analysis of Selected Motor Tools in Children." The findings applied to the science of growing elementary age children, which was sparse at the time; it also identified critical motor skills for kids. In addition, their study revealed all human skills need to be trained during the growth period of 1-to-12 years of age if maximum levels are to be achieved. Bob and Paul Ward used a 16-millimeter camera, an empty track, and a bunch of little kids.

"A lot of weekends, he would just pack up me and my friends and just take us to the park and let us play, and he'd measure what we were doing," said Bob Ward's youngest daughter, Erin. "We would run and jump and run and jump, and every time we thought we were done, he would say, 'One more thing!' And 'One more thing!' It was always 'One more thing.'"

The kids would run fast on the track. They would jump high to touch the sky. They would leap into a sand pit. With a stopwatch, a video camera, a tape measure, a yardstick, a notepad, a pen, and a calculator, the brothers recorded all of the kids' performances.

"I felt like we lived at those tracks," his oldest daughter, Shannon said. "He would use us for his assignment, and it was fun for us. We grew up in that environment, and we didn't know anything else."

This was a planned graduate course research experiment on a bunch of elementary age kids playing at a local school that eventually he would apply in the NFL. Only these findings in Indiana nearly blew away in the wind.

Ward was compiling all of his research and preparing it before computers – via typewriter. He kept his dissertation in a box. One spring afternoon in Bloomington, where tornado strikes are not totally uncommon, a warning came on the television that a storm was coming. The Wards, with the family dog on a leash, were huddled around the TV, waiting for instructions on what to do next. Ward had his dissertation in the box, firmly clutched under his large biceps. The forecaster said if the TV goes white, it's time to take cover immediately.

"What am I going to do?!" Ward nervously asked.

The TV went white.

"Dad ripped up the carpet in the bathroom," his daughter Erin said. "Then, he put the box in the bathtub, and the carpet on top of it."

The storm never hit, and the paper was fine.

By the time Ward had arrived back to Fullerton Community College in the '70s after completing his doctorate, scientific research on athletes was well under way in Eastern Europe. The Soviets and Eastern Bloc countries would test kids from a young age to predict what their potential physical ceiling was and would then put those who were at the top of the food chain in their elaborate and sophisticated training programs. The more radical researchers as well as parents would work on the motor skills of the desired sport from the time their child was an *infant* – and it would usually work. That would be a case of extreme "Tiger Mom-ing."

In the U.S., measurement was in its infancy – it focused primarily on the track and field events, but even then, the research and testing was primitive compared to the Soviets. The U.S. track team would simply pick the three fastest runners, and that was about it. Projection played no part in anything. "When I got involved everybody was starting to look for an edge," Disch, Ward's eventual research partner, said. "And the edge was prediction. Not, 'What could they do?' but 'What will they do?'"

Men such as Bob Ward, Paul Ward, Tom Tellez, Dr. Gideon Ariel, and many others began to study and research U.S. Olympic track and field athletes such as the sprinters, jumpers, and throwers. The technology used to measure was, compared to today's standards, big and crude, but it was an improvement over the rudimentary devices of the previous day.

One of the men who planted a seed in Ward's brain about this was Dr. Ariel – one of the most important sports scientists in the history of the field. Gideon, a grad student at the University of Massachusetts, helped Ward with Dr. Stan Plagenhoeff's biomechanical computer program called "Monster" – Plagenhoeff was one of Ward's mentors. The program was

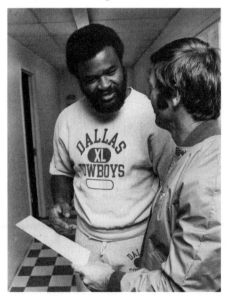

designed for the IBM computers of the day. It used a key punch card, and the Monster's stack was two-feet high. Ward would have to feed the card into the IBM Monster, "When I fed the cards into the IBM computer, the computer felt like it was 'Alive,'" Ward remembers.

Dr. Ariel, a highly regarded PhD in Biomechanics, was so internationally esteemed that he once appeared on *Late Night with David Lettermen*. He worked with Ward on the same USOC Research Team before Ward went to the Cowboys. He related his knowledge

Dallas Cowboys Hall of Fame offensive tackle Rayfield Wright working with Bob Ward in the late '70s.

of the use of biomechanical measurement intended for the Israeli army. In 1968, Dr. Ariel invented the first accurate rapid computer to quantify Olympic athletes' movement. It used a 16-millimeter camera, which then processed data into computer language that could determine what the athlete was doing. In addition, Gideon did the first NFL biomechanics study for Ward on Hall of Fame offensive tackle Rayfield Wright. Rayfield had an injured knee and Ward wanted to determine, biomechanically, what he needed to have Rayfield rehabilitate to improve his in-game performance.

Ward was already with the Cowboys when he still had access to the sophisticated software he had used while working with the USOC's Elite Throwers program. The program, which had been originally developed by the defense department, was used on what is now known as the Internet. The primary function was to provide communication in case of a nuclear disaster where all communication ceased to exist; the Internet would allow a select few computers to continue "talking to each other." This capability simply allowed for faster research and a more rapid exchange of ideas. Today, that's usually called email.

All of the research Ward and many others both in the U.S. and abroad were doing was in an effort to determine what the human body could do and can do in order to reduce the staggering amount of error involved in evaluating human performance. Once Ward took this research to the Cowboys and the NFL, it would grow into a massive business and such a widely practiced field that it has become a seamless part of any major sports organization.

• • • •

By the time Bob Ward arrived with the Cowboys, the team's relationship with IBM was already well established. The team used IBM to chart and categorize college players to evaluate and rank them for the Draft. Equally important inside the giant computers that took up nearly an entire office room on another floor in Dallas was the ability to track and chart what every team did during every single play. What another team did, the Cowboys tracked and computerized. It helped establish tendencies, weaknesses, and gave the Cowboys a major advantage for more than a decade.

"They could chart every play and enter it into a computer, and it would print out all of the plays from the previous game," former Cowboys safety Cliff Harris said. "The Steelers would play the Patriots the previous week and the book the Cowboys would give us would have all of those players. It would have every formation from every play in every situation. They had every route the receivers ran. It had everything, and it gave us a tremendous advantage."

The Cowboys had pages of the following on their own team and opponents: coverages by formation, variation summary, plays by formation and motion, game analysis summary by formation, formation by down and distance, stunts by formation, fronts by formation, and on and on and on. When absorbed correctly, which is not a given, such information can be the difference in the biggest plays of a game, or even a season.

What provided the Cowboys such a tremendous advantage in terms of game preparation was slowly negated by the '80s; every team in every sport, down to junior high football, does it now under the title of "advanced scouting," or sometimes an "analytics department."

The more integrated and cheaper computer technology became, the more sports added to their programs. By the early '80s, Major League Baseball teams began to heavily rely on computer analysis; as a rule, baseball is a far more linear and an easier game to quantify and measure. It's a more "station to station" game, more than hockey, basketball, or football.

In the early '80s, the manager of the Chicago White Sox was an ex-lawyer that, like Cowboys coach Tom Landry, believed there was a major edge to be found in numbers and charting all of those numbers. Tony La Russa, who managed the White Sox from 1979 to 1986, won a World Series title with the Oakland A's and St. Louis Cardinals and is often credited as the manager who fully merged baseball with a spreadsheet.

Noted managers before him, such as Earl Weaver of the Baltimore Orioles and Sparky Anderson of the Cincinnati Reds, started some trends that were based on more computer-based matchups that would later completely dominate baseball. There were others, such as noted mathematician Bill James and former A's general manager Sandy Alderson as well as his successor, Billy Beane, whose forward thinking about numbers in sports was part of this revolution. La Russa is often credited with basing an entire game around matchups and positioning players at certain spots on the field against a particular hitter to a degree that had never been seen before. People did it before him, just maybe not at the electronic level he did. La Russa managed for four decades and was inducted into the Pro Baseball

Hall of Fame in 2014; a case can be made he is the best manager in baseball in the modern era.

Alderson and Beane are the men most associated with *Moneyball,* a term that since the publication of the book has become a verb in sports. La Russa used it long before it was a word.

In football, Tom Landry was Tony La Russa.

"We were already fairly computerized, but what Bob Ward did was to take it to another level," Harris said. "At the time when he got to the Cowboys, the NFL would not allow computerized screens in the press box where the coaches sat. Bob wanted to put them in the coaches' box to compare (statistics) during the game. He ran it through me to the coaches. I went to Coach Landry with it and he liked the idea; it was Bob that got me to do that. It was very innovative. It was math."

It would be virtually impossible to find a computer that doesn't have a mind-numbing amount of data in a coaches' box today in nearly any sport. Football players now use iPads on the sidelines to review previous plays during a game.

One of the more confounding concerns for any coach in the '70s was how to review an opponent before a play began – what formation, schemes, and personnel are the opponents using successfully? By the mid-'70s, all of the teams could easily review this by watching game film of every team. There was no way to do that during an actual game.

In 1977, the Polaroid One Step camera was first produced. This small device would transform modern day photography, right down to the NFL. Polaroid was developed by a man named Edwin H. Land, who left Harvard University before completing his degree in 1926 to work on his own research around light polarization. In 1943, on vacation with his family, Land conceived "instant" photography. Land would eventually develop single-package cameras in the '60s, but the creation of "One Step" brought pictures to life immediately. No longer did people have to take their film to a developer and wait to see what they had.

The pictures were not of a high resolution or a great quality, but they were instant. People could see a photograph – a small square of roughly 4 by 5 inches – in their hands in a matter of seconds. This invention gave Ward an idea: What if the Cowboys used this camera from the coaches' box to take pictures of the game as it happened? A picture would allow the Cowboys to look at what the other team was doing during that *specific* game and make adjustments according to the development of *that* game as opposed to previous games.

Head coach Tom Landry liked the idea. A picture was taken via Polaroid instant camera. To make the walk down between the coaches' box and the sideline took too long, so the team installed a wire between the sidelines and the box and would slide the Polaroid instant shots down to the coaches on the sidelines where players could review them.

That was the very first step to in-game instant analysis and adjustment. As photography evolved, teams would use better pictures to examine everything. The need for a Polaroid didn't last long, however, and the new film that could print pictures from video provided information much more quickly. As photography evolved, teams would use better pictures to examine everything. Today, all of the photographs are available almost immediately; teams can stream video of replays instantly and use computer-operated drones to film practices as well.

• • • •

Statistical analysis and numbers-based breakdowns had been addressed by the Cowboys prior to Ward's arrival in 1976, but he was convinced there was more work to be done and more information and more advantages to be had with a computer.

Dr. James Disch was already a professor at Rice University in Houston in the field of "prediction" when Bob Ward gave him a call. At his core Disch is an economist, something that sports in the modern era has now embraced. Economists can crunch numbers to predict almost anything. Disch was a good friend of Bob Ward's younger brother Paul Ward; the brothers were close while at Indiana.

"Bob is a sports scientist, and at that time, he had nobody to talk to about what he wanted to do," Disch said. "My area of expertise was prediction. I told him to send me what he had; he would bounce ideas off of me and just ask me, 'What can you get from this?'"

Ward's early work and research and analysis of the 1976 and 1977 Dallas Cowboys measured what he could – speed, height, weight, strength. When he measured a player's weight, he didn't just plop him on a scale. He put him in water since hydrostatic weighing is a far more accurate measure of weight and muscle mass. Ward could get a much better reading of a player's body fat percentage through these means.

One of the first things Ward measured for the Cowboys wasn't how much a player weighed when he worked out, but rather what he weighed when he practiced. It is one of the more mystifying practices in sports – players are measured in shorts and a t-shirt rather than standing in their gear and wearing their shoes.

Football players are layered with an array of heavy gear that slows them down and makes them a bit heavier. Ward weighed all of it, from the helmets to the socks. He found that your average player carries 20.8 pounds; today, that figure has been dramatically reduced as companies have continually found ways to make equipment lighter. Back then, Ward's recommendation to players was simple – condition in your football gear.

One of the limitations for Ward was that the technology was only so good. For the Cowboys, he would set up the same type of 16-millimeter cameras he'd used back at the Bloomington, Indiana, tracks to watch his kids run and jump. Ward would set up cameras at certain intervals with lights to measure a player's time in a 40-yard run. They also used strobes to capture multiple pictures as quickly as possible. It was advanced for the '70s, "I loved doing that because Bob made it a competition," former Cowboys linebacker Thomas "Hollywood" Henderson said. "He had that thing set up so you would constantly try to beat the lights."

Perhaps no team in the NFL stressed running more than the Cowboys. And no conditioning coach stressed sprinting over running more than Bob Ward.

"I was up there one time in the late '70s, and Rayfield Wright [Hall of Fame right tackle] must have run the 40-yard dash seven or eight times in a row," former Houston Astros strength and conditioning coach Dr. Gene Coleman said. "He looked at Bob and said, 'Bob – in this organization, when you slow down, you are off the team and outta the league.'"

The players *wanted* to beat the lights. The more they ran, the more Bob measured. The more he measured, the more he could determine.

Ward was one of the first men to implement parachute-training on NFL players – the idea of strengthening through negative resistance. "I was the one holding the parachute on [quarterback] Danny White," said Dr. James

Stray-Gundersen, who worked with Ward on several projects and is widely regarded as one of the most prominent men in his field in sports research and anti-doping policies. He once worked on NASA projects as well as for the U.S. and Norway Olympic teams.

"Bob had an idea to see what a football player could do cardio and endurance wise, and we set up these energy equations for all of football. It was all so much fun then. Some of the wide receivers wanted me to try to get them to out-sprint them."

Ward had one set up where he would put a player on a performance bike and then attach people to it. The player would run 40 yards to generate more resistance; he would measure that. Rather than just measure a player running a 40-yard dash from a standing start, he measured them when they were at top speed. When he measured players lifting from a bench press, he also measured how quickly he could lift as well as how much.

Bob, along with some friends, also measured the game for what it is – a lot of standing around. It's based on quick, explosive, violent movement, and split-second reactions.

At first, there was only so much he could record and determine. He could only test his own players. The first sets of tests were to establish a baseline of sorts, a standard.

The second year, he could actually do some compare and contrast of the players to see where they were and get a better idea of what the genetic code was. Ward could look at a picture of a player's parents and guess a few things.

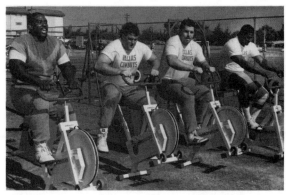

Dallas Cowboys offensive linemen at training camp on stationary bikes in Thousand Oaks, California, in 1987. All of the players are pulling up the bikes to simulate wheelies.

But, once he could extensively test them, then he had a better idea of their ceiling.

There are two distinct schools of thought on the genetic code. One is you can't beat it; the code will determine what you are and how good you are. The other says once you know the code, there are ways to improve it. Regardless, Ward believes most people's potential is determined by the time they're 13.

There is conclusive evidence, rooted again in Eastern European research, that if you train someone from the time they are an infant, you can trump the genetic code; it requires a tremendous amount of work, and repetition. By the time a person reached Ward, either at Fullerton Community College or the Dallas Cowboys, everything had already been pre-determined. It was a matter of maximizing what he had to work with and doing it over and over and over again.

"The idea is to find out what the player is doing and relate everything to the game performance – *that* is analytics," Ward believes. "To determine what resources are required in the game, to do what you need to do."

In his first three full seasons with the Cowboys, Ward determined the only way to increase value in measuring a player was to establish a series of physical tests based on the needs of the position. The same tests he advised the Cowboys to use in 1979 look almost identical to the drills the NFL uses with prospective rookies in the Combine every single February.

For years, the Cowboys were renowned for their ability, and money, to sign more than 100 undrafted football players every spring in an effort to find that one guy who every other team missed. After coming up with a handful of tests, Ward knew by noon of the first practice how many of these rookie hopefuls could potentially join the team by training camp.

At the end of the third year, the players and the team were well-versed in Ward's research and testing methods. Across the board, players found they were growing stronger and faster. Measuring the specifics of a player's time in the 40-yard dash, allowed Ward to find holes in a runner's stride length and minute places to improve. The same was true for strength and for hitting.

"What Bob found out was all of these tests, they didn't predict who could play, but they could accurately predict who could *not* play," Disch said.

By figuring out who could not play, Ward created a massive opportunity that every team would eventually seize. The more quickly a team or a coach can figure out who has the talent, the more time can be given to the players who can actually *play*. "What Bob did so well through this was to determine and to develop training programs to maximize the potential of every athlete,"

Disch said. "You are not going to have 45 super stars, but you can maximize every one on a team."

After his third season, Ward realized what he had been studying and researching was not necessarily wrong but had missed the essence of what sport is – it's about the game. This decision was based on the analytics derived from analyzing all the data he collected on players. How a player does on a test or in a drill may not be an accurate reflection of how he will do when the boat hits the beach. It's no different than a basketball player doing drills. It's no different than a law student. The aspiring lawyer may be great in the classroom and ace the bar exam, but turn out to be a complete failure in a courtroom. There had to be a better way to evaluate players than what he'd been doing.

"It's on the field," Ward clarifies. "It's in the game. The only way to really do it is measure them in the game while they are playing. While the fans are cheering. While they are tired or stressed – how do they perform in the game. That's the work and the study that matters."

Ward would continue to test and evaluate players in practice and in the weight room based on camera and computer study for the rest of his career. The type of testing and research he did in the late '70s on the Cowboys when they were running, jumping, lifting, or standing is now so common that a person can do it at a local fitness gym.

He would take what he'd found and then try to measure the players in an actual game.

• • • •

A bigger, albeit quieter, element in the history of sports-related analytics is injuries. One of the most underappreciated elements to Bob Ward's tenure with the Dallas Cowboys was the infrequency of injuries. Whether this is a coincidence, players playing hurt, or the combination of his research with his training programs is impossible to know, but players who worked under his care all said they never sustained major injuries in his time; that the rash of injuries that so frequently hits NFL teams in the modern era was not an issue then.

In the early '80s, he wrote a 23-page report that summarized a variety of football training models and studies on certain areas of the game, most notably injuries. He listed the frequency of injuries. In order, they were:

knee, strain fracture, foot-ankle, contusions, misc., head-neck, shoulder, hip, wrist-hand, and elbow. There is no mention of "concussions"; although it is a safe bet that one of football's most controversial injuries of the modern era was classified as "misc." in Ward's tenure.

What Ward found was that the players receiving fewer injuries were those players who:

1. Reacted Faster
2. Faster Footwork
3. Better Agility
4. Better Speed/Endurance
5. Greater aerobic capacity
6. Higher percent lean body weight
7. Younger
8. High grades for games played
9. Slower in 40-yard sprint

Ward's conclusions suggested things that are in direct contrast to the accepted attributes of a football player. Coaches covet speed often as much as any other physical attribute, but the faster player is hurt more frequently.

Research similar to this led companies to continually strive to make equipment lighter and better. Pads used today in hockey and football, as well as other gear, are so good and so sophisticated and so light they bear little resemblance to what the players of the '70s and '80s used. As to their effectiveness in reducing injury, that can be debated. The numbers say players are more apt to be injured today, despite the advances, than in Ward's era. But is it because players take themselves out of the game more now for fear of injuring themselves, or because the collisions are more violent?

As much as Ward tested, he wasn't able to test everything. Ward and Stray-Gundersen wanted to conduct echocardiograms on the players, a test that produces a visual display of the heart's activity as a way to find out if a person has a heart disease or is vulnerable to heart failure. "Sudden death in sport is obviously a very important issue, and we were unable to conduct that test," Stray-Gundersen said. "If you do an advanced screen, you can pick out the people that are likely to have that happen to them."

A few years after Stray-Gundersen and Ward wanted to have this test done on Cowboys players, this very issue was brought to national attention.

Loyola Marymount power forward Hank Gathers was the nation's leading scorer and rebounder in NCAA Division I basketball, and it was assumed he would be one of the top picks in the coming NBA Draft.

In December of 1989, he collapsed while attempting a free throw during a game in Los Angeles. Tests later revealed he had an abnormal heartbeat, so he was prescribed medication. Gathers felt the medication was affecting his play, and during a game on March 4, 1990, after completing a dunk, he was on his way back up the floor when he stumbled and fell. He died on his way to the hospital. Reports said later he had cut back on his medication. Since his death, the need to diagnose an abnormal heartbeat has only intensified.

In July of 1993, Boston Celtics All-Star shooting guard Reggie Lewis collapsed during a light workout in the Boston-area. Shortly thereafter, Lewis died of cardiomyopathy, something the test Stray-Gundersen and Ward wanted to conduct could have revealed.

The problem is sometimes a player simply does not want the test because he does not want to know the result. In 2005, the Chicago Bulls traded 7-foot-1 center Eddy Curry, even though the team selected him with the fourth overall pick of the 2001 NBA Draft. While with the Bulls, tests revealed Curry had an irregular heartbeat and a heart condition similar to Hank Gathers. The Bulls wanted Curry to take a genetic test, but he had no interest.

The New York Knicks traded for Curry with the agreement that such extra testing would not be included. Curry would play seven more NBA seasons for three more teams; the heart issue would not be an issue. He just wasn't very good.

• • • •

In the mid-'80s, Ward had an exchange with a computer software man who proposed to meet with Tom Landry and a few coaches to pitch a plan that would, on average, be worth an average of seven points per game for the Cowboys. The proposal was called "Game Theory." The man who invented it was named Jeff Sagarin.

Later, Sagarin would go on to develop a ranking system that would make him widely famous in sports. His programs have been used by the NCAA men's basketball selection committee, and he is routinely listed in *USA Today* and other prominent media outlets. To sports fans, "Sagarin Ratings" require no explanation.

In 1985, when he made a pitch to the Cowboys, he wrote:

"Suppose you are the DEFENSIVE team and you think you 'know' the OFFENSIVE team's tendencies for the situation in question. Our methods can then be used to rank (from best to worst) your defenses against the OFFENSIVE mix. As the DEFENSIVE coach, you would use the defenses which make the GAME VALUE to the offensive team as low as possible."

What Sagarin outlined was a fairly complex formula for a team to pick plays based on a ranking system and tendencies that had been tabulated by previous games.

"Given tendencies," Sagarin wrote, "our mathematical method (IN FACT, THE VERY SIMPLEST APPLICATION OF IT) can be used to 'price out' or rank your own team's plays from best to worst, depending on DOWN-DISTANCE-FIELD POSITION situation."

The program Sagarin outlined and pitched sounds very similar to the models used by the wildly popular EA Sports video games, known as *Madden NFL* – or commonly just referred to as "Madden."

Despite his pitch, and Ward's endorsement, the Cowboys never hired Jeff Sagarin.

• • • •

When Bob Ward reached out to Dr. Ralph Mann, the pair had figured out that their studies of guys working out in a gym or even on a practice field had some promise. They also agreed this was the only way to go. They began to film games and try to measure the players from footage. "It was absolutely archaic the way we did it," Mann said. "We would put cameras at the top of the stadium and try to pan around to catch everything we could. It wasn't high-resolution like they have today, or anything close to it."

Before a Cowboys game at the Superdome in New Orleans, Mann and Ward would haul a bunch of heavy equipment to the top of stadium. They had as many as five large cases in their haul; the Superdome didn't feature elevators, so the pair just climbed to set all of it up. "I was younger than Bob so he 'let me' carry it," Mann said jokingly.

When the game was over, they would review the videotapes of all of the players to measure what they did and how well they did it. They would break the tape down, frame by frame, to see what they could find. "We looked at everything we could possibly think of," Mann said. "Take a position on the field, and we tried to measure it. How quickly a player could move, how fast a player was, how hard a player hit."

The results said virtually no player ever hit their maximum speed on any given play, including a wide receiver running a straight line; they have too much to think about and process to run at top speed. "They are maybe 85 percent of what they can run," Mann said. "It's the same for any human being – give them a complex task, and the brain has to process it, which slows us down. They have to worry about where the defender is, where the sideline is, where the ball is, and all of that prevents him from reaching maximum speed.

"It's not about who can run the fastest, but who can run the fastest with a lot on his mind."

They also found that a running back's speed was not as important as his quickness. How fast a running back could "hit the hole" – reach the target his offensive linemen created for him – was as important if not more important than the player's end-to-end speed.

Unlike a baseball statistician who can simply plug in numbers based on a myriad of variables, what Ward and his buddies were doing required far more time and effort. All of this research and input was exhaustive and took months to complete in an effort just to build a single set of standards. There was no quick turnaround.

"We were delving into the same kind of thing as *Moneyball*," Mann said. "The *Moneyball* thing was a smart statistician that said you have to find what really matters. We were doing the same thing, only we had to create it. *Moneyball* is based on situations and men on base, and those are easy to find because they are right there. What is not easy to find is how fast someone is running down a field with all of these other players running around. It's chaos."

Collecting this type of in-game information, combined with the data collected on the players in a weight room, gave Ward a clearer idea of what each player could do. All of this – *all* of it – is now common in today's era of sports. Men such as Mann and Ward and a few others set the baselines, the minimums, and the standards for all others. Once they gathered enough numbers and enough data and set up enough scenarios, then they could come up with the rest of the "equation." They could come up with their hypothesis and then test it on-the-field.

In the mid-'80s, these two created an on-the-field analysis system that measured all of what a player did while he played the game. "It gives you a better handle of things, and it gives you a handle on who is busting it out there and who is dogging it," then Chicago Bears head coach Mike Ditka said of the new technology. "You could look at it along with an existing player and see the intensity level that he played with at the start of the season compared to the end of the season. ... We can cure the physical part, if it's mental then we have to look at what we are doing as coaches or get new players."

Today, thanks to lighter, cheaper, and better technology, the type of on-the-field research and analysis Ward, Mann, and Disch were doing is everywhere. Technology, such as Global Positioning Satellites (GPS), has allowed for measurement of nearly everything with an exactness that could not exist when Ward was with the Cowboys. Software called "Zebra Systems" tracks everything an NFL player does in an NFL game, which breaks everything down to the smallest decimal point to be consumed by players, coaches, and even fans. They're measured for impact, driving force, acceleration, and overall running speed.

All of this information and statistical analysis is as much a part of the fabric of the sport as a helmet, a sock, or a weight rack in every single sport. It affects the way teams build rosters, draft players, and prepare for opponents. Players now expect and demand it. In 2015, Portland Trail Blazers forward LaMarcus Aldridge was a free agent meeting with prospective teams to decide where he would sign his next contract. In his meeting with the Los Angles Lakers, it was reported that Aldridge was turned off from the team because they didn't stress the analytics of basketball.

"It truly is amazing to see this term 'analytics' and what it's become," said Dr. George Kondraske, who met Ward shortly after he became a professor of bioengineering at the University of Texas-Arlington in the early '80s. The men conducted several studies together, and Kondraske bounced his concept of "Performance Theory" off Ward; it's a cause/effect theory based on the necessary elements of a successful player.

"People were doing it long before it was called 'analytics.' But it's become chic, and now it's hot. In reality, analytics is multiple things, and in the future it could be completely different. The basic idea is to have data and then to develop a model based on that data."

Ward and Mann knew they had hit on something when they broke down the performer *as* he performed. They also knew they were looking for a needle in a stack of needles, but to find it looking at the game was the best method of research. "The demands of each sport are so specific and the complexity so high that any attempt to evaluate an athlete in any manner outside the actual on-field environment is an exercise of futility," Mann wrote in a paper titled "On Field Analysis."

"Bob really was one of the innovators I tried to emulate," Mann said. "We had such a good time, and he really left a mark on football. Half of the people don't realize how important he was. Everything he was doing back then, they take for granted now."

The ironic part is that despite this reality it has not stopped anybody from trying to evaluate athletes on something outside of the game. Mann wrote there were six variables that are involved in the development of an athlete, nearly all of which could be measured and quantified. It illustrates the inherent difficulties that come in predicting success for an athlete or a team:

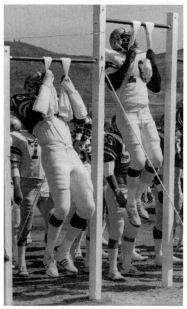

Bob Ward had the Dallas Cowboys use towels on pull-ups to improve grip strength. Ward believed if you could keep your grip while lifting, then you could make the tackle in the game.

1. **Physical Development Level**: Early physical developers have an advantage when competing with athletes their own age. This quickly disappears when everyone reaches maturity. Likewise, late developers don't reach their potential until much later, which shifts their performance peak much later in their career.

2. **Coaching**: The coaching an athlete receives, whether good, bad, or non-existent will make a major impact on their development process. An individual with good coaching will display more of their potential than those with little or no coaching. Bad coaching may ruin an athlete's potential entirely.

3. **Level of Competition**: Those athletes that are placed in a highly competitive, high stress environment will

raise their performance level accordingly. Likewise, those that are not challenged will not achieve their greatest potential until they move up to a more competitive environment.

4. **Injuries.** Physical issues can easily preclude an athlete from ever having the chance for success. Regardless of the talent level, a major injury can either end a career, postpone it to the point where the success window is missed, or permanently degrade their talent to the point that they can no longer reach their pre-injury potential.

5. **Luck:** There are so many "what if" possibilities where athletes are given chances, then show their talent to an unsuspecting audience. "What if" Tom Brady was never drafted in the late rounds and given a chance to succeed on the field, "what if" eight other alternate golfers hadn't opted out of the PGA Championship so that John Daly could not only play but win the Tournament, or "what if" Michael Jordon or John Elway had chosen baseball over the sport that made each of them famous?

6. **Measurements**: Perhaps the biggest commonly known reason for prediction efforts failing to predict elite level success is the measurement process. For those individual sports where success is determined by time, like track or swimming, the task is much easier (although by no means simple). The most difficult prediction process involves team sports that rely on scoring or measurements that can be affected by teammates or opponents. In these sports, athlete potential is often measured using simple skills that are performed off the competitive field of play. The most obvious example of this is the set of skill tests that are performed at the NFL Combine each year to measure an athlete's strength, speed, and/or quickness. The problem with these kinds of tests, whether in football or any other sport, is that they do not deliver on their predictive goals. Although these tests will determine if an athlete can play the sport, it has been shown countless times that they cannot predict the level of success that the player will achieve.

• • • •

By the time the Cowboys lost their third consecutive NFC title game in 1982, computer technology was well on its way to becoming more widely used in society. Video game consoles were being produced, meaning people no longer had to go to an "arcade" to play a game. The massive computers the Cowboys had in their offices were actually getting a bit smaller. People were beginning to buy something called a personal laptop. Technology was becoming something for the people.

Fan participation in sports, however, remained spectator oriented. Fans just watched. There was no integrated fan participation in an actual NFL, MLB, NHL, or NBA game. Thanks to computers and analytics, the way fans consume sports today is something that Ward only had a minor concept of in the early '80s. At that point, he had seen enough to know that statistics and real-time scoring would eventually be available to fans, but nothing like it has become.

Advanced analytics gave birth to a little nothing called "Fantasy Sports." Advanced analytics helped to create a massive, multibillion-dollar industry and new revenue streams for leagues, teams, and enterprising entrepreneurs. Fantasy sports is the combination of numbers, extensive statistics, and a rather simple mathematical formula that allows fans to play "games" based on the games themselves.

There are stories out there to suggest the first "Fantasy Football" league was actually created by some football fans in Oakland, California in 1963. In 2010, ESPN produced a documentary called *Silly Little Game*, which stated the first fantasy league was actually created by baseball fans in New York in the late '70s. It was called "Rotisserie Baseball," which was based on a restaurant in Manhattan called "La Rotisserie Francaise."

Whoever created it is not getting any royalties. Reports from *Forbes* and the Fantasy Sports Trade Association say that more than 33 million Americans play fantasy sports and help to create more than $4 billion in economic movement. Hotels and resorts offer "Fantasy Drafts" where "players" go for a weekend of fun and drafting their fantasy lineup. It's a form of legalized gambling.

Based on the staggering amount of research they compiled, Ward and Mann have written software specifically for Fantasy Football. Now it's a matter of finding a buyer in a highly intense, competitive, and flooded market.

• • • •

Men like Ward who infused numbers into sports helped to create a massive phenomenon that is now ingrained in sports culture. Before Ward did his work with the Cowboys, numbers were almost exclusively reserved for baseball. Together, they made numbers a part of every sport. Even today, Ward has boxes and boxes full of data and research he compiled on the Cowboys during his tenure. There are so many numbers that even Ward concedes, "We've only scratched the surface on this. I'm not even sure what it all means."

The proliferation of research and numbers has not been well received by everybody in sports. A lot of people believe analytics is a made-up term to create jobs for people who never played. "I've always believed analytics was crap," former NBA player and Basketball Hall of Famer Charles Barkley said in an appearance on the TNT network in February 2015. "It's just some crap that people made up to try to get into the game because they had no talent."

A lot of people agree with Barkley on this because analytics runs face first into change. "This is not just sports, but it's generational," Dr. George Kondraske said. "It is hard to take an athlete, or a coach, at the top of their profession and say, 'This is the science of what you are doing and this is what you need to change to do it better.' They don't fundamentally want to change what they are doing."

At its core, analytics is simply about information and "getting the meaning of the numbers." The more information in anything is better, but there must exist a medium between what the computer finds and what the eyes see.

"What we are going to see is, if we have not already, is the coaches coming up integrate them both equally," Dr. James Stray-Gundersen said. "There is no way a highly successful or highly-trained athlete does not use [analytics]. Back in the days when we were first sorting this stuff out, it did give us an advantage. The people who did it ended up winning. Pretty much everybody else saw it and said, 'I guess we have to do this.'"

• • • •

Al Vermeil is the only strength coach to ever win titles as a strength and conditioning coach in the NFL and NBA; he did with the San Francisco 49ers in the '80s and the Chicago Bulls in the '90s. Not long after he took the job with the 49ers, he visited Ward and the Cowboys to see what he should be trying to implement for his new team. A couple of years later, Vermeil's 49ers defeated Ward's Cowboys in the NFC championship game.

Vermeil agreed with Ward that all of the science and research is helpful, provided the person in question ask and answer the following: "Can he play?" meaning, is the player any good? "Does he have instincts to play the game? Can he play the game?"

The worst answer to these questions for any position coach or strength and conditioning coach is, "No – but if you work with them."

"No, he can't," Vermeil said. "When I was with the Bulls, we were looking at this kid [before the start of the NBA Draft] who could run forever. He could sprint. He could jump out of the gym. But he could not play. He was not a player. I never tried to determine if a guy could play. I tried to determine [for the Bulls before the Draft], 'This is physically what he can do to play.' I can't make him rebound or play defense. You cannot put anything there that intuitively is not there. The key is to get good players, and Bob helped the Cowboys do that. That's it. If you are having a drag race between a Ferrari against a Volkswagen, the Ferrari is going to win every single time.

"You want to know why I won Super Bowl rings and NBA championship rings? Because I had Joe Montana and Michael Jordan. If I don't have those guys, you don't know who the hell I am."

Bob Ward was not dumb enough to believe his methods and research made Roger Staubach a brilliant passer or a Hall of Fame quarterback. He simply gave Staubach the resources and programs, based on statistical research, to make him a more physically fit athlete. That is why analytics is so valuable and, today, so widely accepted. It is about finding the information to put a person in the best position to be at their best in every possible scenario.

What Bob was doing then made him an outlier. Today, he's an inlier.

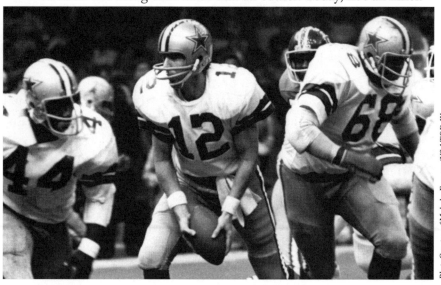

Super Bowl XII –Dallas Cowboys quarterback Roger Staubach taking the snap against the Denver Broncos; the Cowboys went on to win 27-10. Bob Ward simply gave Staubach the resources and programs, based on statistical research, to make him a more physically fit athlete.

CHAPTER **9**

PANNING
FOR GOLD

*"First get your facts, then you can
distort them at your leisure."*
– Mark Twain

Bob and his family learned quickly: Being a part of the Dallas Cowboys in Dallas, especially when they win, is loads of fun. The Cowboys, along with the New York Yankees, are the biggest name in professional sports. To be associated with the Cowboys was to enjoy a degree of celebrity status, which Ward and his family enjoyed.

As a football player who never quite reached the pinnacle to which he'd aspired, Bob Ward was well-versed in the success of the Cowboys by the time he took the job in Dallas. Los Angeles had the Rams, and further down the road was the San Diego Chargers. So, as someone who lived and worked in Southern California, America's Team was not a priority until they were his priority. By the middle of the first season in 1976, he quickly realized why they were so good – the coaches and a sincere commitment to winning. The Cowboys spent big money to win, to find players, and to make those players better. Nearly everywhere Bob looked in his weight room, there was another guy who could play.

In football parlance, "to play" is not just a regular verb. Some players are "just a guy," meaning they are not especially noteworthy. When a guy is good, it is important to emphasize the word "play," in verbal italics: He can *play*.

The mid-to-late '70s Dallas Cowboys were stacked with guys who could *play*.

One year after winning the Super Bowl against the Denver Broncos in 1977, the Cowboys were a meager 6-4 with six games remaining in the season. Despite their vast talent, they were barely above average. From that point on, Nov. 12, 1977, they were dominant. They won their final six games of the regular season, only one of which was closer than seven points. In the playoffs, they were equally dominant and won the NFC Championship game 28-0 against the Rams in Los Angeles.

It set up one of this sport's most memorable games – the Dallas Cowboys versus the Pittsburgh Steelers in Super Bowl XIII in Miami. That game ranks as one of the best in league history for the simple fact it featured 14 players who would eventually be inducted into the Pro Football Hall of Fame, not to mention head coaches Chuck Knoll and Tom Landry and other team executives. Las Vegas oddsmakers had the Cowboys as 4.5 favorites to win their second consecutive Super Bowl.

With the Steelers leading in the third quarter 21-14, the Cowboys moved the ball to within 10 yards of a touchdown. Quarterback Roger Staubach spotted wide-open tight end Jackie Smith, who had come out of retirement to play for the Cowboys for just one year, in the end zone. The ball was there, but Smith dropped it. The Cowboys had to settle for a field goal.

The Cowboys lost 35-31.

The play sadly defined what was a brilliant career. Google "Jackie Smith" – one of the first phrases to automatically pop is "dropped pass." The cruel irony is that Smith was renowned for not dropping *anything* before that moment. Prior to being a Cowboy, Smith played the first 15 years of his NFL career with the St. Louis Cardinals and was a five-time Pro Bowler. He extended his career for one additional year specifically to play for the Dallas Cowboys, so he could have a shot at the Super Bowl.

He was 38 when he came to Dallas, and everybody on that team wanted it for him. He had labored in obscurity for a bad Cardinals team, and this one season was his best chance. Unfortunately, by the time he came to the Cowboys, he was finished. He'd had a total of eight catches in the previous two seasons combined. With the Cowboys during the 1978 regular season, he had no receptions at all.

In the playoffs, however, he had three catches including a touchdown. But, in the Super Bowl, the *one* time Roger Staubach threw his way, Smith dropped it for one of the most famous plays in Super Bowl history. Even after he was inducted into the Pro Football Hall of Fame in 1994, the play continued to shadow Smith.

Had Smith caught the ball for a touchdown, there's no guarantee that the Cowboys would have won.

Ward was with the coaches in the coaches' box. "No one could believe Jackie had somehow missed the catch," he remembers. "A couple of coaches screamed and yelled. In the locker room, no one wanted to add to his misery by talking to him. After all, what could you really say to him? Then, we went to the party after the game with the coaches, the players, and the wives, and no one talked to Jackie. Everybody felt so badly for him. You could tell it was just tearing him up."

• • • •

The Cowboys were loaded with players who could *play*, but sometimes that's not enough.

There was no team any better in the NFL at finding guys who could play than the Dallas Cowboys. There was no team any better at evaluating, ranking, and cultivating NFL talent. This franchise set the standard. It did not take Ward long in his job to learn the lifeblood of any professional sports franchise – the Draft and player acquisition.

After he figured it out, draft preparation became another area where his fingerprints would remain absolutely indelible.

"When we talk about Bob Ward – he didn't even know it, but he created an entire industry in what he did," said former Dallas Cowboys strength and conditioning coach Joe Juraszek, who worked for the team in the 21st century as well as at the University of Oklahoma. "Those guys back then, and Bob was a huge part of it, created an industry solely based on preparation."

The Dallas Cowboys did not invent player evaluation at the college level, but they certainly perfected the process. In the '50s, Cleveland Browns and later Cincinnati Bengals founder Paul Brown was trying to evaluate player speed. He came up with a distance of 40 yards as a valid measurement since that was, and is, about as far as a player would need to run on a given football play.

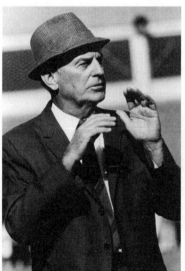

Legendary Cleveland Browns and Cincinnati Bengals head coach Paul Brown – In the '50s, he came up with a distance of 40 yards as a valid measurement of a player's speed.

Photo Courtesy of Malcolm Emmons/USA TODAY

The 40-yard dash remains the gold standard of evaluating the speed of an NFL player. The distance remains unchanged, but its relevance is now often debated, lamented, and criticized. There is a cadre of people in the NFL who feel this length is not applicable, while there are those – Pro Football Hall of Fame executive Bill Polian for example – who believe this distance is an accurate measurement of a player's speed on special teams, i.e. punts and kickoffs. Regardless, the 40-yard dash is a physiological measure that has existed for decades. Just as the bench press has to measure a player's strength. The high jump. The vertical jump. The shuttle run. Name a basic exercise you performed in elementary or middle school gym class, and those remain "physiological measures" used to determine what the body can do in a football game. That will never change, even if it should.

What Paul Brown did to measure prospective players for the NFL, the Cowboys did to organize and transform scouting and player evaluation. In the '60s, the Cowboys devised a "grading" system that basically remains in place today. It was a way to assemble all the potential players into a giant system and draft according to an assigned ranking. This grading system, which was later computerized by a subsidiary company of IBM, is often cited as the reason the Cowboys became one of the most successful football franchises in the '70s.

The grading system merits mentioning because the men devising it – Cowboys head coach Tom Landry, Cowboys vice president of player personnel Gil Brandt, and Cowboys team president Tex Schramm – are often credited for transforming professional football.

"Truthfully, a lot of the stuff we did, Paul Brown had already done," Gil Brandt said. "The difference was when we did it. He was the first guy to give the Wonderlic test, but he did it after he signed the guy or drafted him. We did it *before* we signed him or drafted him."

The Pro Personnel Evaluation System was a collection of observations and assessments of a player by a member of a front office. Each player was assigned a numerical grade. When the following chart was made, the NFL Draft was 12 rounds. It is seven rounds today.

The following is the grading system the Cowboys created. The number on the left represents where the player is projected to be drafted; the number on the right is a numerical grade a scout assigns to the player in an effort to assess and quantify the person's ability and projected production.

PRO GRADE

1/1: 99-90: Unusual. Pro player without weaknesses. Super star, pro bowl player. Will start immediately.

1/1 & 1/2; 89-80: Very good. Pro player without weaknesses. Has pro bowl ability. Should start during his rookie year.

2/2 & 2/3; 79-70: Good. Pro player without weaknesses. Dependable, steady player. May need a year but will be able to start his second year.

3/3 & 3/4; 69-60: Above average. Pro player without weaknesses but has inconsistencies he must overcome in order to be productive for a contender. May be a conversion to another position; may not have progressed because lack of experience, small college exposure, played another sport, late growth, immaturity, or some other reason brought out by the scout in the report. Could have been hampered by injuries. [Here, scouts must ask themselves, "Do you think he will overcome inconsistencies, or will he have them as long as he plays?"]

5/6 & 7/8; 59-50: Average. Pro player who has one weakness in his characteristics. May be overachiever but be limited in ability. Could have reached his potential; could have overcome his weakness or play in spite of it. [Scout must determine potential in evaluating these players.]

9/10 & 11-12; 49-40: Below Average. Pro player with more than one weakness in his characteristics. Has to overcome weaknesses and inconsistencies. Normally a late [draft] choice type player but scout may see better potential in his evaluation. [Some good players come out of this category by overcoming weaknesses and inconsistencies. They may overcome some and play in spite of others.]

Rookie Free Agent (undrafted): Doubtful. Pro player with more than weakness in his characteristics. Free agent type. Usually has size only. Must have something that warrants bringing him in.

TC 20-29: Barely. Sometimes goes to camp to fill a late need.

RJ 10: Never. Reject.

When each player has been assigned a grade, they were then placed into a different evaluating system:

BLUE: 10.0, 9.7, 9.5, 9.3, 9.0

A great player who dominates the game at his position on a consistent basis. A blue player will be true "Pro Bowl Caliber" year in and year out. A blue player will be able to lead his team to the Super Bowl. Examples – Barry Sanders, Jim Kelly.

Sanders was the third overall pick in the 1989 NFL Draft and is widely regarded as the best pure running back in NFL history. He is a member of the Pro Football Hall of Fame.

Kelly was the 14th overall pick in the 1983 NFL Draft by the Buffalo Bills. He played 11 NFL seasons, led the Bills to four consecutive Super Bowls, and is a member of the Pro Football Hall of Fame.

RED: 8.9, 8.7, 8.5, 8.3, 8.0

A very good player who demonstrates consistent production. A red player will be a consistent factor in winning games for his team and will definitely be one of the top players in the league. Examples – Tim McDonald, Ken Harvey.

McDonald was a second round pick of the St. Louis Cardinals in 1987 and played 13 NFL seasons. He started 187 games and went to six Pro Bowls.

Harvey was a first round pick of the Cardinals in 1988 and was a four-time Pro Bowler in 11 NFL seasons.

GREEN: 7.9, 7.7, 7.5, 7.3, 7.0

A solid, steady player who is good enough to start. He will make a positive contribution toward the outcome of a game. He has production. Examples – Lance Smith, Ricky Proehl.

Smith was a third round pick of the St. Louis Cardinals in 1985. A guard, he played 12 NFL seasons with two teams and started 165 games.

Proehl was a third round pick of the Phoenix Cardinals in 1990, and he did not retire until after the 2006 season. He played for six teams and caught 669 passes for 8,878 yards and 54 touchdowns.

GOLD: 6.9, 6.7, 6.5, 6.3, 6.0

Should be a backup player. A gold could be an older player on the way down or a younger player on the way up. A gold could be a starter, but in that case, you would definitely be looking to upgrade, unless he's a young ascending player. Examples – Danny Villa, Ed Cunningham.

Villa was a fifth round pick of the New England Patriots in 1987 and played 12 seasons for four teams.

Cunningham was a third round pick of the Phoenix Cardinals in 1992 and played five seasons, starting 47 games.

PINK: 5.9, 5.7, 5.5, 5.3, 5.0

A younger player who has developmental qualities and should ascend, but has limited playing time. Examples – Rob Baxley, Jeff Christy.

Baxley was an 11th round pick of the Cardinals in 1992; he played one NFL season and a total of six games in 1992.

Christy was a fourth-round pick of the Minnesota Vikings in 1993 and would go on to enjoy a 10-year NFL career. He was a starter for nine seasons.

"When we did this – there was no form to it. Nobody had a form, so we just created one," Brandt said. "We had to establish a grading system."

For the men trying to perfect this process, they approached it like McDonald's restaurants.

"What McDonald's did was to create a system that measured everything, right down to when the cars would come by and what time of day and how the area of that restaurant was going to change and grow," Brandt said. "They had numbers for everything to determine if that site was going to be good for one of their restaurants." The Cowboys did the same only with players.

This system was not and is not foolproof. Teams routinely grade players whose future performance far exceeds the expertise of veteran scouts, analysts, team executives, and more specifically, the ranking of a computer. That is why there are "busts" and "surprises" in every draft class, which makes the process so fascinating.

In 1998, the San Diego Chargers selected Washington State University quarterback Ryan Leaf with the second pick of the NFL Draft. He went on to personify "bust"; he played two seasons with the Chargers before he was released. He played in four games for the Dallas Cowboys in 2001 and was done with football for good. In 2000, the New England Patriots selected University of Michigan quarterback Tom Brady in the sixth round of the NFL Draft. He since went on to become the most successful quarterback of this century with multiple Super Bowl wins.

There is no exact, foolproof method to nail this crucial inexact science to the success of any professional sports team, but the Cowboys' grading and organizational system changed professional football.

By 1979, this system was well in place, and Bob Ward was well into conducting the studies and the research with which he would eventually become synonymous. The draft, and more specifically player evaluation, was an area of particular interest. What he did in 1980 was devise a way to gauge evaluation and measurement of players even further.

"What the Cowboys and Gil Brandt did to scouting and player evaluation in the 1960s, that is exactly what Bob Ward did to strength and conditioning when he came in to the NFL in the 1970s," said former Dallas Cowboys and Denver Broncos wide receiver Butch Johnson. "That's how big of an impact he made."

• • • •

On January 11, 1980, Bob Ward sat in his office and completed a formal seven-page memo to Cowboys head coach Tom Landry. Ward simply titled it, "1979 Draft Analysis." Ward would never know what Landry, Tex Schramm, or Gil Brandt ever did with this study, but years later, it is apparent this memo made it somewhere high in the Cowboys, or even NFL, offices.

Ward applied a program called "Discriminant Analysis" after the 1979 NFL season to determine if certain variables were accurate in predicting whether a player would make it in the NFL. His test subjects were the entire 1979 draft class. Ward used statistics and a wealth of data to assess these players' performance over the season. There are some similarities to Ward's memo and the system the Cowboys were using, but there are some findings that were a revelation, and a revolution.

Describing his findings, Ward says, "Grades given by scouts and the athletic ability considered separately from scouts had a 69 to 75 percent chance of determining whether a guy would play in the NFL."

Then Ward wrote down something that would eventually become a staple in the NFL. The best predictors for each position:

Tight End/Offensive Line (75 to 86 percent chance of correct selection)

Scout, 5 yard burst, 20 yard, 40 yard, arm span, lean body weight, clean bench press, squat back, vertical jump, standing long jump

Defensive Line (86 percent chance of correct selection)

Pull up corrected, standing long jump, height, audio reaction, total body reaction, foot reaction, agility

Defensive Back (100 percent chance of correct selection)
Scout, 5 yard, 20 yard, 40 yard, arm span, clean, bench, squat back, vertical jump, standing long jump, backpedal 30 yards

Wide Receiver (93 percent chance of correct selection)
Scout, 5 yard, 20 yard, 40 yard, arm span, lean body weight, clean, bench press, squat back, vertical jump, standing long jump, agility, foot reaction, height

Quarterback (83 percent chance of correct selection)
Height, agility, foot reaction, 40 yard

Ward also factored in "Cultural Determinants" of prospects, meaning a player's family, with whom he associated, and other individuals the guy called friends. Ward also tried to weigh in what type of person the prospect was – a loner, gregarious, sensitive, or idiosyncratic. The entire concept was rooted in reducing error by adding more variables to quantify the statistics, something that professional sports would later completely marry. By the time Ward wrote this memo, he was advocating and pushing for as much statistical analysis as computers could manage.

One day during practice, Tom Landry and Bob Ward were chatting about computers, mainly Bob's prodding for more computers and more technology.

"Bob – we already *are* computerized," Landry said.

"Coach, no we're not," Ward said.

Ward knew that, while the Cowboys used computers and data analysis to break down game film and apply to game preparation, there was so much more potential to be had. He recommended more new and more advanced prediction equations, more testing, and the addition of psychological measures.

As Ward was learning, exposing someone to new information that could help was one thing. Getting them to do something with it was a much harder proposition. By 1980 with the addition of Bob Ward's insight, the Dallas Cowboys clearly established they knew what they were doing in regard to draft preparation and player acquisition; they created a formula that other teams would mimic and use with great success.

In 2015, it is evident that the memo was not thrown into the trashcan.

• • • •

By the summer of 1982, as computers became more common in society, Ward had a clear vision of how sports would look in the 21st century. He saw it all coming. In the article he wrote for the June-July issue of the *National Strength and Conditioning Association Journal* titled, "Superconditioning Technologies For Sports in the Twenty-first Century" he covered the future of the NFL Draft:

PLAYER SELECTION – DRAFT

"College recruiting and NFL Drafting techniques of the twenty-first century will use Biomechanical analysis to measure the ability levels of prospective players during the actual game. Physiological measures as taken today will pale in significance when compared to actual game data. This is the future, because anything other than game data is a poor reflection of reality."

The amount of data and statistics to grade, evaluate, and quantify in 1982 is almost nothing compared to what a team, or just a mere fan, can use today.

In 1982, a running back was "evaluated" based on how many yards he gained, his yards per carry average, the number of catches, touchdowns, etc. Roughly, a player was assessed on about five or six numerical categories. In 2015, the amount of statistical data a running back can be judged and evaluated on can be paralyzing. A running back's yardage is now broken down by "yards after contact" – meaning how many yards he gained after he was first hit. The yards can also be broken down by the formation the offense is in, the direction of the run, etc.

A quarterback's accuracy is now broken down by how far the passes travel as well as how many yards were actually gained not by the pass but by the receiver after he catches the ball and advances it on the field.

Back then, there was nothing called *Pro Football Focus* – a hugely popular website that gathers an array of information that fans, teams, players – and player agents – use to quantify a player or a particular performance.

This wide array of data collection is not at all unique to football; it applies to every single sport. Baseball's use of biomechanical analysis is simply classified under the catch-all title of *Moneyball*. It's created a business and ostensibly opened a massive new avenue in that sport that many could argue has been a boon for a game that has never surpassed football in terms of its national popularity. It has revolutionized player evaluation, something Ward was so far ahead of that only a limited number of people realized he was the first who brought it out of the Olympic sports and took it to the NFL.

What has changed since the early '80s is the measurement and analysis within those activities to see how or if the body can improve those basic standards. It's not just about running the 40-yard dash, but instead figuring out where the runner is accelerating, stride length, and more specifically, how to improve such individual elements.

It is in this measurement, research, and analysis that Dr. Bob Ward made perhaps his biggest discoveries and impact on professional football: the micro versus the macro. Ward did not believe that the 40-yard dash should be applied across the board to all players. For linemen – the biggest players on the field, he thought the more applicable measurement for speed should be no more than 20 yards. Having played football, Ward thought the majority of the emphasis on training for a football game should be on powerful speed, or explosiveness.

This is the oddest part where the relationship between the game, the physiological, and the biomechanical do not always line up scientifically, mathematically, or even close to perfectly. The challenge was, and remains, to balance what the eyes and experience saw versus what the data collected and quantified.

"The most important criterion, and maybe the most overlooked, is the ability to play the game," Ward acknowledges. "There should be no equivocation on this point."

Ward knew then just as everyone in high major sports understands that, sometimes, the gut should trump the spreadsheet. What Ward wanted to do, however, was to teach the gut different instincts when looking at a player.

"On paper some players look All-World but on the field look All-Thumbs," Houston Oilers strength coach Bill Allerheiligen said in the October-November 1982 edition of the *National Strength and Conditioning Association Journal*.

Ward wanted to weed out the "All-Thumbs" players before their in-game issues ever became a problem for the Cowboys.

The process of player selection and player evaluation as a means to determine what a player is, can, and will be remains forever maddening, confounding, absolutely essential, and eternally compelling because of its unpredictability. This is where a team, your team, improves or dies. This is where the 36 inches are so essential, now more than ever before. This is also where men like Ward, and countless others, run into one of the biggest problems in their chosen profession. Getting someone, or something, to change can be an inherently impossible task.

It is also in this area where some of his work, and specifically some of the things he wrote in that 1980 memo to Tom Landry, remains so everlasting.

• • • •

The last place anybody should want to be in mid-February is in central Indiana. Indianapolis in the winter is not exactly a tourist haunt. It is cold. It is eternally gray. The sun has flown south for the winter. Regardless, for about one week, it is the epicenter of all things football. In retrospect, why the NFL picked Indianapolis, Indiana, to hold its glorified tryout and meat market for its latest round of prospective employees is mystifying, other than its central geography on a United States' map.

The NFL Combine was originally called the National Invitational Camp (NIC), and it was first held in the far more moderate climate of Tampa, Florida. It had 163 college players. Then, the NIC moved to New Orleans for a couple of years with one year in Arizona before it moved permanently to Indianapolis in 1987, where it has been ever since.

"It really wasn't that big of a deal," Ward describes. "You just had us all there, and we'd talk to players. We would work them out and talk to them. It really was nothing special, but it was just a place where we could all go."

The purpose of the Combine was to put everybody in the same spot in order to provide the teams opportunity to meet prospective players up close. It was part meet-and-greet and part skills exhibition. Scouts and coaches met with the players. Players would provide their medical history to teams, and then they would be measured (height/weight) and tested in a series of drills. It was informal, rather disorganized, and somewhat quaint where everybody could move freely in downtown Indianapolis without the burden of much of anything.

No one in the media covered it because nothing happened.

"It's funny – now it's this big deal with all of these people and fans," said Pro Football Hall of Fame member Mike Ditka, who was the head coach of the Chicago Bears when the first organized Combine was held. "In the beginning not every team was even there."

That reality itself is unfathomable. Today, there is the Senior Bowl and multiple other occasions when teams can send representatives to meet prospective draftees. If it sounds like overkill, it is. There is nothing more overkill about the NFL than player evaluation, specifically the NFL Combine. "Back then, not everybody had bought into the idea. Some teams just didn't do it," Ditka said. "Now, every team and *everybody* is there."

The destination for this "event" is reflective of the NFL itself – it was sitting on the edge of a massive expansion, of becoming the most popular sport in North America. By 2015, the NFL Scouting Combine has become the "event" after the Super Bowl, complete with press credentials and live television coverage on the NFL Network. In 2015, the NFL announced 1,000 press credentials were issued, and now, everything is organized and structured down to the minute. Multiple websites cover just player evaluation and many NFL "Draft Experts" to narrate the events.

All 32 NFL franchises send their entire personnel staff from coaches to scouts to general managers to the owners themselves to Indianapolis for about one week. Teams spend hundreds of thousands of dollars to staff an event that, ironically, many coaches loathe. It has become another seven-figure NFL event, only this time, not much actually happens. But you *have* to be there.

For the players themselves, it is one of a handful of glorified interviews they could have with a prospective team to land one of a few highly coveted jobs. Every NFL team features a roster of 53 active players, each making over six figure salaries. The competition for these jobs is mercilessly tough, and savagely cruel. The amount of money involved in the NFL allows for cost overruns to be routinely ignored. There is virtually no, or minimal,

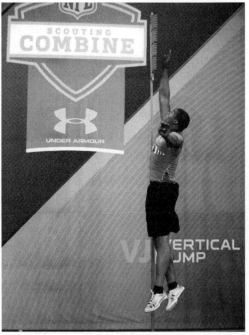

The NFL Scouting Combine puts everybody in the same spot in order to provide teams the opportunity to meet prospective players up close and see their skill set. Here is Cam Newton at the 2011 NFL Scouting Combine. The former Auburn quarterback was selected with the first overall pick in the 2011 NFL Draft by the Carolina Panthers.

Photo Courtesy of Brian Spurlock/USA TODAY

incentive for teams to check their expenses because the revenues are so high. When it comes to player evaluation and scouting, teams spend millions to staff countless college games during the season, every bowl game, and the host of college postseason games, which include the Senior Bowl, the East-West Shrine Game, the Medal of Honor Bowl, and the National Bowl.

And representatives from teams will routinely talk to college coaches, assistant coaches, and the players themselves many times before the Combine itself. And then they talk to them again at the Combine. And then they talk to them again at the player's "Pro Day," which usually consists of the same drills on their respective college campuses.

And then, after the Combine, before the NFL Draft, teams will fly those same players they have already talked to ad nauseam to the headquarters in Indianapolis, Green Bay, South Florida, or any other NFL city. All of this is put under the "collecting information" umbrella.

"There are way too many people involved today," said Gil Brandt, who has been around this for more than four decades and remains active at the Combine. "By that I mean there are too many people and too many voices [within an organization]. If you take 10 people and send them to the same restaurant, some will say, 'That is the best steak I ever had.' And another four will say, 'That's one of the worst steaks I ever had.' And you listen to all of them because they all have qualifications and credentials.

"It was so much easier and better to formulate an opinion of what a guy was when there were just two or three guys doing it. The offensive line coach would want you to draft seven offensive linemen, and the linebackers coach would want six linebackers. You have to eliminate those voices."

Because the event is so big and has become such a staple of the NFL calendar, players routinely drop out of college immediately after the season ends specifically to work out at facilities and with trainers who are preparing them for this "event."

It is no different than spending money to take a prep course for an SAT, LSAT, GRE, or any other major entrance exam. Trainers are paid by agents to prepare clients for the NFL's test – the Combine.

The whole idea is to not just pass the test, but to ace it. Yet, it is littered with inaccuracies, beginning with the most basic essential – these are a series of tests for football players who in this environment are not wearing football gear. The NFL Combine is often called the "Underwear Olympics" for this reason.

In an effort to quantify a player's, as Ward wrote, "Physiological measures", the NFL adopted a series of six events for the Combine that would ostensibly reflect a player's innate athleticism. They are as follows:

1. The 40-yard dash
2. Bench press
3. Vertical jump
4. Broad jump
5. 3 cone drill – the cones are set up in an "L" shape. From a starting line, the player runs five yards to the first cone and back. Then, he runs around the second cone, and then he weaves around a third cone, which is the highest point of the "L," changes directions, and comes back to the second cone and finishes.
6. Shuttle run – the idea here is to test lateral quickness and "explosion in short areas," as defined by the NFL. The player starts in a three-point stance, runs five yards to his right, touches a line, retreats 10 yards to his left, left hand touches the line, pivots, and he turns five more yards to complete the drill.

"The Combine? Those drills, those *exact* drills – those are the exact same ones we did when Bob Ward came to the Dallas Cowboys [in 1976]," former Dallas Cowboys wide receiver Butch Johnson said. Johnson played for the Cowboys from 1976 to 1983 and for two additional seasons with the Denver Broncos.

"There was no Combine when I got into the league. There was none of it. And when the Combine started, what things were they evaluating guys in? The same stuff Bob Ward had us doing when I was with the Cowboys. The stuff you see today – and he will never get the credit – is what he brought into the league. It's a little different, but not much."

Unlike today, where there is sophisticated precision timing equipment as opposed to a hand held stopwatch, most of this is rooted in tradition. All of this is about the "Physiological measures" Dr. Bob Ward suggested to determine what the player can do, athletically speaking.

"That's really about what it is. You see all the time guys perform really well at the Combine and then they don't turn out to be what 'They are going to be,'" said Cincinnati Bengals starting quarterback Andy Dalton, who was a second round draft pick of the Bengals in 2011. "As a quarterback, it does not matter how you run, but it's how you throw it and just because you do well at a combine, it does not mean you can read a defense. That's why after the Combine, you do private workouts for teams. They want to see how smart you are, how much the game matters to you, all of that. The Combine is to show athletic ability and that it can translate to the game. If you perform at the Combine, you really need the tape [the game film] to match it up."

Now for the ironic part – the vast majority of people who are paid handsomely to attend and work the NFL Combine will all tell you the same thing – it's not worthless, but it's not necessary. And they don't like it.

"It has been the standard for so long that coaches and outside people train athletes to be combine proficient," said former long-time NFL strength and conditioning coach Joe Juraszek, who also worked at the University of Oklahoma. "I mean, I was guilty of it, too. I could choreograph and count out the steps in some of those drills and reduce a guy's time."

New England Patriots head coach Bill Belichick reportedly is not a fan of the Combine because, he feels, nothing the potential draftee does in the workouts is a good indicator of what he can do on the field during an actual game. Because there is so much money on the line, players will spend hours preparing for these specific drills. Athletic trainers, employed by agents, are employed year round at notable training facilities in Phoenix, San Diego, and North Texas to work with players specifically with one goal in mind – to kill it at the Combine.

In 1995, Boston College defensive end Mike Mamula would become everything that is inherently problematic about the Combine. Mamula was projected to be drafted in the third round, but his "draft stock" took off after he excelled at the Combine. His name is synonymous with the Combine and "busts."

He had trained with a professional trainer for months for the events, and when it was time to take the tests, he killed them all. The Eagles selected Mamula with the seventh overall pick of the 1995 Draft, and he went on to play six seasons, start 64 games, and collect 31.5 sacks with one defensive touchdown. If he was a second or third round pick, his name would not be part of NFL lore. But it is specifically because of how well he did at the Combine and how that performance in a series of drills influenced the Eagles' decision to make him a first round pick that made him famous.

"You *have* to watch the game," Ward always says.

In the game, Mike Mamula was good at Boston College. In his pre-NFL workouts, he was outstanding.

Some players even believe the Combine, and training for it, actually works against rookies in their first year in the NFL.

"You are working on leaning down. You are working on straight-line speed. You are working on endurance in lifting," Dallas Cowboys center Travis Frederick said, who was a first round pick of the team out of Wisconsin in 2013. "In football, generally you strength train in lifting. Short yardage bursts, short yardage change of direction and quickness. Those types of things. I wouldn't tell [potential] rookies to do anything different. They pay people a lot of money to make those decisions for them and to help guide them through process. The Combine has become such a big deal that you have to train for the Combine. I think that's a slippery slope to decide which one you are going to train for."

There is little reason *not* to change the NFL Combine, but given its success, there is zero incentive to alter a single thing other than to expand it, and sell tickets. Knowing that, there is an industry of trainers whose professional existence lives on this event.

Veteran trainer Brian Weese prepares his clients for the NFL Combine with the following:

"The first thing I tell the guys when they get there is, 'You are going to be treated like a world class track athlete. Forget everything you know about football,'" he said. "You are breaking them down and looking at extreme minutiae and what it takes to be better at that test. I tell the boys every year, 'There is football season and there is Combine season.'

"Combine performance, there is no other animal like it. There is nothing in sports like it. When you are training a football player for a season, you have certain needs. Strength and power – they apply themselves to their team sport. But, when you train for the Combine, none of what you are doing with the football player that will be drafted, none of [the Combine] preparation is rationally usable in the world of football."

With so many professionals on the record saying the system is flawed, why doesn't it change?

Despite the many advances men such as Dr. Ward and so many others have made in their respective field and the crushing amount of analysis, data, and information available, changing the way a person thinks, or a league continues to conducts its business, is an entirely different animal.

It comes down to not what the body has done in terms of statistical production in a myriad of potential scenarios, but what the body can do in terms of raw performance. And actual game data should always trump the physiological, but it some times does not.

For better or worse, back in 1980, Bob Ward had no idea what he would help create.

Ward's Words
My Bloodline Might Make it to the NFL

Self-admittedly, I would have liked to play pro-football. I tried to continue my football playing career after Whitworth College and the Marine Corps, but it was not in God's plan. My tryouts with the New York Giants and B.C. Lions of the Canadian Football League both ended up with me being cut, in part due to injuries. I made it further than most when it comes to playing football, but not as far as others.

Maybe my genes will make it further.

My grandson, Taylor Symmank, is a senior punter-kicker at Texas Tech University, though he didn't learn to punt until he was in college. Taylor had been a very good soccer player at a high school in McKinney, Texas – not too far from my house in Dallas. I had seen him play enough soccer to know that the ability to kick was there; it's like anybody I had ever worked with – find the right skill for his talent and unleash it. Once Taylor learned the mechanics of punting, he has been brilliant.

I was a pretty good athlete in high school and in college, but I was nothing like Taylor. He's a punter, but he probably could have played other positions had he wanted to. He can do things I certainly could never do.

As a senior at Texas Tech, Taylor was clocked running the 40-yard dash at 4.4 seconds. The fastest guy on the team ran a 4.32. I'm not sure I could do either of those times in my car. The best vertical jump on the team at Texas Tech was a defensive end named Zach Barnes, who hit 36.5 inches. Taylor's vertical jump was just one inch shy of that mark.

Punters are better athletes today than ever before. Take Steve Weatherford, for example. He has had a long NFL career as a punter, most recently with the New York Giants, and is well-known for his all-around physique and athleticism. Taylor is like that. He can do anything, he just happens to be able to punt the ball a long, long way. A lot farther than his grandfather ever could.

It's fun to read about him asking the new players on the team to race him. They all think they can beat him because he's the punter. It doesn't end well for them.

Before his senior year at Texas Tech, Taylor was named the Big 12 preseason punter of the year. I'm hoping he can do what his grandfather could not and make it to the pros as a player. Personally, I'm hoping the Dallas Cowboys sign Taylor to an NFL contract.

CHAPTER **10**

FOOTBALL FROM MARTIAL ARTS TO THE UFC

"Learning is never cumulative, it is a movement of
knowing which has no beginning and no end."
– Bruce Lee

Bob Ward had been with the Dallas Cowboys a little more than a year when he rolled out the creative, innovative portion of his personality and brain to his test subjects, more frequently known as human beings. The Cowboys players looked at Ward as an ally, an asset, and trusted that he had their best interests at heart. Many of them also understood their conditioning coach, while fully committed to his job, was not fully committed to remaining with it long term since Ward still had an attractive tenured teaching and coaching position at Fullerton Community College waiting for him.

The players were concerned if the Cowboys did not do something about it, Bob Ward was going back to California. Not every player was familiar with the inner working's of Bob's family life, or that Bob's wife, Joyce, was actually itching to join him Dallas. What they saw, however, was Ward's non-office office still exposed to the "great outdoors" – more specifically a hot Texas sun.

Safety Charlie Waters came to work one day and looked over at what he feared was an exhausted Bob Ward. Ward's face was overly red from the sun, and the man simply looked tired. "If we don't do something about this, we are going to lose him," Waters said to no one in particular in the locker room. "We've got to keep him."

Ward was not the type of person to threaten his boss or exercise anything as a means of leverage. Those traits are not in his personality. In his mind, if the Cowboys wanted him to stay, they would make that readily apparent. Around the time Waters made this comment to no one, team president Tex

Schramm got Ward a real office with a real roof at the practice field and the weight room. This and similar little "gestures" made it increasingly more difficult for Ward to want to leave.

Also, in the offseason of 1978, Ward found that necessity is still the mother of invention when it comes to everything, including sacking opposing quarterbacks. With the help of an old friend, Dan Inosanto, Bob Ward introduced the world of Bruce Lee and martial arts to the NFL – a pairing that actually endures to this day.

• • • •

At its core, football is violent, full of impacts, collisions, and crashes. The game lends itself to injury, sometimes life altering.

"You are a Pro and have to play hurt," Tom Landry would often say.

What Bob Ward saw in the '70s when it came to players playing hurt or injured was nothing new to the sport, then or now. "A minimum twice a year, I was knocked out cold. I mean – *cold*," Waters said. "I know for a fact I went back into games when I had a concussion. Most of us did. I was a professional football player, and by God, they paid me to play football, so I was going to do everything in my power to keep playing football."

If that meant playing hurt, so be it. If that meant playing injured, that was OK, too. Team doctors across the NFL routinely applied pain-killing injections to players all in the name of getting them back on the field. "It's an indictment on sports for sure, that doesn't make it right, but it's what we did," Ward explains. "You stress the necessity in a strength and conditioning program to develop tissue strength to avoid injury, but in many instances, that's a losing battle."

Ward remembers what it was like to be knocked out. When he was playing for his high school team, he was knocked out by an opposing player named Louie Elias. Coincidentally, Elias went on to play football at UCLA and in the CFL and would later enjoy a long career as a Hollywood actor where he appeared in the original *Star Trek* TV series as well as the first *Charlie's Angels* series.

Between his experience and his research, when Ward was with the Cowboys, players recognized whatever he was doing would work.

"There is no way of proving this, but I am convinced some of the stuff he had us doing in terms of conditioning and things like that are the reason we never got hurt," said former Cowboys offensive lineman Brian Baldinger, who was with the Cowboys from 1982 to 1987. "In my first three years in Dallas, we never had a major injury. No ACL tears. No hamstrings. We practiced just as hard as anybody in the league, and we never got hurt. All of the different stuff he had us doing, it all strengthened your bones, your forearms, your shinbones. It all helped."

This doesn't mean everything Ward taught was a foolproof way of preventing injury. He certainly had no control over what a player did when he was on his own, outside of the Cowboys' facility. Football, like most sports, is filled with young men in the prime of their physical lives who are amped up, competitive, and believe they will win… forever. It's also a game rooted in machismo culture that was often counter to what a guy like Ward knew to be correct.

"It was like the water deprivation thing that coaches used to do. I used to see guys take muscle relaxers, shoot up painkillers," he recounts. "I took a muscle relaxant one time, and I absolutely hated it. But I wasn't a player. Back then, guys did that stuff because they didn't know or they didn't care."

Concussions were not much a concern then either; players got their "bell rung" and returned to the game ASAP. In the modern era, after extensive study and research, there has been new information to suggest that to do so has left former players with disastrous mental and physical consequences. There have also been a slew of lawsuits against the NFL, one of which resulted in a controversial class-action settlement that approached $1 billion.

There is currently new technology being tested to prevent players from playing with concussions while also monitoring the activity of the brain to allow for a quicker return. If a player fails certain concussion-related protocols, most leagues now have rules in place stipulating they are out for the game.

"Now they can determine what part of the brain is concussed," Dr. James Andrews said. "If a certain part of the brain is concussed, there is certain rehabbing you can do whereas we used to say, 'He's out for a week.' Now, they can put them through rehab and it depends on what part of the brain was concussed. They are able to figure it out."

The NFL continually adding more rules, ostensibly designed to improve player safety, is not a new trend. This has been going on since 1962. Long before concussion-prevention became a topic of concern, and the need to prevent potential damaging litigation costs arose, professional football had been slowly trying to eliminate dangerous plays to the head. Whether the reasoning was because of potential lawsuits or merely an effort to reduce violent plays, pro football has been aware of these hits for decades.

- In 1962, the AFL/NFL banned intentional grabbing and shaking of facemasks.
- In 1974, the NFL banned intentional blows to the helmet with a player's hands.
- In 1977, the NFL banned the "head-slap."
- In 1980, the NFL applied a 15-yard "personal foul" penalty to any player who directly strikes, swings, or clubs a player in the head, neck, or face.
- In 1996, the NFL banned helmet-to-helmet hits.

Long before the NFL became mired in concussion-related litigation from retired players, the league at least was semi-aware that there were some things on the field that had to be banned. That while no one had published the documented evidence of long-term effects to the head and brain potentially from football, the appearance of some techniques in the sport were too dangerous to even watch.

When the NFL outlawed the "head-slap" – a move that had been the dominant defensive technique for decades – it was a blow for defensive players of that era. Have a friend hit you in the head three times in the span of three seconds and see how well you do. Hall of Fame defensive end Deacon Jones is synonymous with a particular head-slap move that could potentially be devastating for an opposing offensive lineman. In fact, Jones is credited for inventing the term "sack" – a tackle of the quarterback behind the line of scrimmage. He was elected to the Pro Football Hall of Fame in 1980 after a career where he was voted all-NFL in six consecutive seasons and made eight Pro Bowls.

"The head-slap is a vicious move," Deacon Jones said in a 1980 interview; he died in 2013.

"They outlawed it because I could break a man's neck. And I guess they didn't want those sissies nowadays to get their necks broke."

Jones was known for hyperbole, and for promoting himself and his considerable achievements. When Jones would break down his movements, he would slap an opposing player with right and lefts to the head. Then he would take his knee in an attempt to hit the player in his stomach. "That's the killer," he said. "You gotta to do the 1-2-3 – it's like a dance step - *boom!*"

Like Bruce Lee's Cha Cha Cha. The Cha Cha Cha rhythm and its variations are used in football as well as in virtually all other team sports.

Once the league made this move illegal, defensive players had to find something to remain as effective.

"The other thing you have to remember is that back in those days, a guy could wear a 1-inch pad around his forearm. So it didn't hurt to head-slap a guy," former Cowboys receiver Butch Johnson said. "The helmets were thinner then. A guy is wearing a 1-inch pad around his hands and forearms; he hits a guy with a cross shot to the head, and he's gone for the game. And you wonder why there are so many concussions."

• • • •

Although it was out of his title as conditioning coach, as a former player and a source of endless curiosity about sports, Ward made it a mission to find a different method for defensive players to negate the loss of the head-slap. This need took him back to Whitworth and to Los Angeles – to one of three men trained by internationally renowned martial experts Bruce Lee.

Thus, Ward's idea to incorporate martial arts into a football player conditioning was part curiosity and part necessity to the players and coaches. But Ward's USMC and martial training knew a "Applied Martial Arts Program" was a simple decision. Maybe it could work. "I thought he was crazy," said former Dallas Cowboys wide receiver Butch Johnson, who arrived to the team when Ward did.

Around the same time Bob Ward was playing around the beaches in Southern California, Dan Inosanto, a nationally recognized 20th century martial artist, was raised in the poor region that is Stockton, California. He was athletic, and he played sports all day long with a particular passion for track and football. He was fast – he ran a 9.5 in the 100-yard sprint in college. And he could run forever, but his problem was his size. He was small. He was almost too small for local high school team football. During Inosanto's time in high school, the school needed a new football coach, and one elderly gentleman was looking for a job, at least on a part-time basis.

The local high school gave Amos Alonzo Stagg a part-time job coaching the football team. Stagg is considered the founding father and pioneer of American football. He founded the American Football Coaches' Association in the '20s, and among some of his inventions for football are the tackling dummy, the huddle, the reverse play, a man in motion, knit pants, putting numbers on player jerseys, and naming a play by a number or numbers; he also invented the awarding of letters to football players.

"I didn't know who he was, other than people talked about him and that he was very famous," Inosanto said. "He coached the punters, the kickoff people, the conversion people, and the special teams – which I was one."

During every football practice Amos Alonzo Stagg coached the short Filipino-American. This is akin to learning baseball from Abner Doubleday, basketball from James Naismith, or driving a car from Richard Petty.

"He taught me how to hold the ball and do the kicking game," Inosanto said. "I really don't think until I was out of college and out of the military service I realized who this guy was. I didn't know that Amos Alonzo Stagg was such a big deal or that he was considered one of the fathers of football. I really just knew he was there every day at our practices, and, really, he was much more than a football coach to us. He was a personal coach to me."

Like Bob Ward, Inosanto found his way to Whitworth College from California. He was a freshman with Ward's younger brother, Paul, when Bob Ward was a senior at the school in Spokane. Inosanto knew Bob Ward at Whitworth for just one year, but the man made an impression. Near the end of his freshman year, he was assigned his final term paper for his English class— the subject he chose was Bob Ward. Inosanto received a "C" for grammar, but an "A" for content.

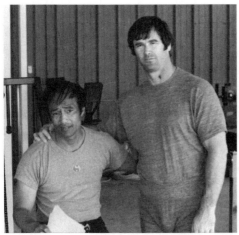

"Bob was an absolute hero of mine," Inosanto said. "I idolized him. He was such a good athlete. He was the first one to introduce weight training to us – not many people did that back then. He created the course outline and taught the first weight training physical education course at Whitworth. But he had this way about him that made you look up to him. I really wanted to *be* him."

Bob Ward with friend and Bruce Lee disciple Dan Inosanto, who worked with the Cowboys on introducing martial arts, at the Cowboys' facility in Dallas in 1978.

The two fell out of touch after Ward graduated from Whitworth; Inosanto continued his college career there where he ran track and played football. After graduating, he, like Ward, entered the military. During his time at Whitworth, and more so in the military, Inosanto started to play around with the ancient eastern practice of martial arts. He had done some as a kid in Stockton, but the more he did it, the more he liked it, and unlike football, his stature was not an issue in martial arts.

By 1964, he was training often and martial art was gaining some fractional movement in the U.S. There was an international championship tournament in Long Beach, California, and the event organizer wanted Inosanto to act as a host of a guest coming in from China. The guest was Bruce Lee. Although born in San Francisco, Lee was raised mostly in China and, by 1964, was well on his way to becoming the single most influential martial artist of any generation.

While touring and guiding Lee around Los Angeles, Inosanto asked Lee if he could train and study with him. Lee agreed; three weeks later, at a martial arts event in Los Angeles at Chinese Theater, Inosanto's role in the demonstration was to be, essentially, the tackling dummy.

"You can be the fall guy," Lee told Inosanto. "I'll teach you how do this."

Inosanto eventually became one of the few people – there are just three – to study and train with Lee. By 1966, Lee had appeared on *The Milton Berle Show* and was on his way to becoming a Hollywood action star. Lee would become one of the most iconic, celebrated, and recognized names in martial arts. He would bring martial arts to the United States in a way no one ever had.

The Inosantos were regulars at the Lee household for family dinners. Lee, who trained in the Chinese art of Wing Chun – more commonly in the U.S. called "Kung Fu" – believed, preached, and taught the necessity to learn everything.

"People usually don't remember, or they don't know, that my godfather [Bruce Lee] was an American," said Inosanto's daughter, Diane, who would later go on to become a Hollywood stuntwoman and stunt coordinator. "He liked American sports."

Around the time that Bruce Lee was making the transition from Chinese action film star to Hollywood film icon, Bob Ward was at Fullerton

Community College coaching track, teaching, and doing the life thing. He was too busy to be bored, but as a constantly curious man, he looked at martial arts and wondered exactly what it was like. From the time he climbed from the crib, he was always moving in an effort to move in a different manner. He had never tried martial arts, other than some boxing and wrestling.

One evening at his home in the early '70s, he called his old friend from Whitworth – Inosanto. At the time, Inosanto was teaching junior high school and teaching martial arts on the side.

"Dan – what would you think about training me in what you do?" Ward asked.

The man who looked up to Ward so much just a decade earlier as his role model was now his teacher. Ward learned martial arts from Inosanto, and was eventually qualified to teach Jeet Kune Do (JKD), Bruce Lee's art. At about this time, Ward was a fit 215 pounds of muscle, but when it came to this craft, size was not the issue. He trained in Jeet Kune Do, but he could never overpower the much smaller Inosanto. Losing has a way of making a believer out of everybody.

Ward learned first hand the benefits of martial arts, which more than a decade later would benefit him in a different job. Before that day, however, on July 20, 1973, Bruce Lee tragically died at the age of 32. He left a massive international legacy on martial arts, on fitness, on Hollywood, and vicariously, his footprint is stamped indelibly in the skills of many other sports; that includes Ward bringing these skills to America's Team, the National Football League, and beyond.

• • • •

When the NFL outlawed the head-slap, Ward picked up the phone again. He had an idea, which at the time was so far-fetched and outlandish that he knew some of the players and coaches were going to think him an outright idiot trying to justify his paycheck with some half-cocked, stupid idea, even though he had been applying his JKD knowledge from Day One with the Cowboys.

"Dan," Ward told him on the phone, "What would you think about training the Dallas Cowboys in what you do?"

"Are you serious?" Inosanto asked. "You want me to train the Dallas Cowboys!?"

Inosanto agreed, and after hanging up the phone, he asked rhetorically – "What does what I do have to do with American football?" Shortly after the Cowboys arrived in Thousand Oaks, California, Ward had Inosanto down to visit as a guest lecturer. It was the first time a pro football team would be exposed to the ancient practice of martial arts.

"What the hell is this guy doing here?" Cowboys defensive coordinator Ernie Stautner asked defensive tackle Randy White before the "course" started.

Like so many things Ward did, on first sight, Dan Inosanto working with football players made *zero* sense. But, on closer inspection, it was completely logical.

"This is why Bob Ward is a genius," Inosanto said, "no one else would have seen how much martial arts is used in a given football play. I never even thought of it, and I played football."

Inosanto walked out onto the field in Thousand Oaks, flanked by the mountains and wrapped in the warm air of Southern California's August temperatures to size his new students. He had worked with and trained students for more than a decade by this point, but this crew was not at all like any of those he'd worked with before. The people he always taught were at least eager, if not always capable or the most athletic. These guys were more than capable, but their interest level varied from interested to distracted to bored. They were all highly skilled athletes who had already perfected their craft of American football, and their previous experience said that was all they needed.

Inosanto had originally wanted to teach the Cowboys what Lee had mastered – Wing Chun. "Wing Chun takes no less than three months. Every day," Diane Inosanto said.

Inosanto did not have three months. He didn't have three days. He had about three hours, if that, to make an impression. If guys were interested, they could see the teacher after class, so to speak. Inosanto decided the Filipino practice of Hubud was the better route with football players. The whole goal was for Inosanto to teach, or at least expose, players to his craft. Hubud focuses more on the hands and has roughly three moves to master. For Inosanto, Hubud was a better use of his time.

Ward wanted to find something to replace the head-slap, and fortunately, this was it. By the new NFL laws, *these* hand slaps and hand rip moves were clean and effective.

"For me, I had to do it," Randy White said. "When I entered the league, my move was to grab [an offensive lineman's shoulder] and to put my arm over. The NFL out-lawed that move. When Bob brought this to us, at first, it was a little crude."

When a play begins, and the collisions start, the primary goal of everyone is to free their hands and use them the way they want or need to "shed" blockers or to slow potential tacklers. After Inosanto's first session with the team, he realized not everyone was buying in. He knew going in he would be met by some trepidation, and skepticism.

"The guys I know who found it useful were the linemen," Inosanto said. "I had several guys who had been wrestlers in high school and in college who said they found it helpful and they saw how it could be helpful and beneficial to them. It was just one of those things that you were open-minded about it, and you could see how it worked."

One of the assistant coaches approached Inosanto after the practice session and greeted him with a masculine but sincere handshake. Mike Ditka was a fan of this, and when he became the head coach of the Chicago Bears and later the New Orleans Saints, he had experts in this area do the same lessons with his teams.

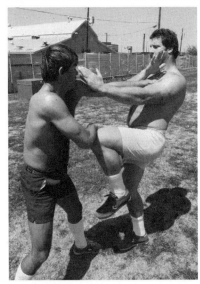

Bob Ward brought martial arts to the Cowboys as a way to improve their style of play. Here he is with Dallas Cowboys Hall of Fame defensive tackle Randy White (right) practicing these skills.

Before Inosanto left Thousand Oaks, he continually stressed one point to every willing pair of ears that was open to his message: "Use other people's energy to your benefit." That sentence is part of a larger message he tried to part to all of the Cowboys:

"The truth in combat is different for each individual in this style:
1. Research your own experience
2. Absorb what is useful
3. Reject what is useless
4. Add what is specifically your own"

Charlie Waters heard this and understood what it meant, but had little idea how to actually apply it. Waters knew at just under 200 pounds that size-wise he was over-matched on nearly every play. He had to do something in order to be able to either move or shed a blocking player. With Inosanto gone, Waters asked Ward what to do when he faced an opposing offensive guard who likely weighed 100 pounds more than he did.

"The first thing you have to do is give them a target to hit," Ward said. "And then, you immediately have to take it away."

Waters looked at Ward as if he was indeed crazy. Ward instructed Waters to expose a part of his chest for opposing offensive linemen to reach for or punch; when the player did that, it would make him off balance and vulnerable. Waters was then to reach for that hand and pull him down. The first time he tried it during practice, he exposed a part of his chest...

"I could not believe it, but the damn thing worked," Waters said. "The guard went for it, and I grabbed him and easily pulled him down."

When Waters watches an NFL game now, he routinely sees similar moves, when people are dumb enough to put themselves in a position to go for it.

"The NFL is a copycat league. It's always been that way," Waters said. "Once they saw moves like that worked, everybody started doing it. It's to the point where guys teach and coach that all the time."

Studies that Ward, Inosanto, and others conducted all showed that the impact of these moves roughly takes about two weeks to grasp and then improve. When White looks back on his Hall of Fame career, White specifically credits Ward introducing martial arts for a good portion for his success.

Safety Cliff Harris – the guy whose first question to Ward was "How can you make me better?" – was sold after Inosanto's visit. Harris' father had been a fighter pilot in World War II and served in the South China Sea; in his time in the service, Harris' father learned Jiu Jitsu and later introduced the craft to his son. When Inosanto began his instructions, Harris was at least somewhat familiar with the practice and some of the moves. He had never thought to use any of it during a football game, either in college at Ouachita Baptist or with the Cowboys. He didn't use it until Ward showed him how.

"Bob was a scientist and I am a math and physics guy; that was the part where Bob and I really related a lot," Harris said. "I related to the motion that he was trying to teach. I was a little guy, and it was my responsibility to make plays all the time on bigger guys. When a play started, a wide receiver would come down and try to stand up to block me. Before Bob taught me, I would just try to run through it or slam my way in there.

"Bob taught me – and I really don't even know how to describe it – this move where the receiver would come at me, and with my right hand, I would push up, and with my other arm, I would swipe them away. And it worked. And I would make the tackle."

Sound a little like "wax on, wax off"?

In the world of football where the margin between winning and losing is normally inches, the slightest movements of the hands can actually make a large difference. When done correctly at the right time, they can make the ultimate difference, which is why Ward's introduction of martial arts to the NFL remains. Martial arts remained a part of the Cowboys' training for the duration of Ward's tenure with the team.

Other teams – notably the Seattle Seahawks, San Francisco 49ers, and Oakland/Los Angeles Raiders – eventually hired Inosanto to consult, and other martial arts people entered the league peripherally as personal trainers.

"In the very beginning, when we were at Thousand Oaks, I know not everybody saw the value in it," Inosanto said. "Bob could see the value in hand trapping. What you are trying to do is to shorten the response time.

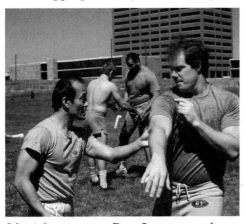

It's all about touch, and that is the value. Honestly, I would not have seen the value had Bob not had me down there to talk to those guys. I would never have thought martial arts would enhance the skills of a football player, but he did and that's why he was so ahead of the game. It really takes just one guy to make a difference, and then he talks to a teammate, who talks to a friend, and on and on. That's why you've seen it become more

Martial arts expert Dan Inosanto works out with the Cowboys in the late '70s in Dallas. Bob Ward was one of the very first to bring martial arts to players in the name of strength and flexibility.

common to the point where you don't even know you are watching martial arts in a football game."

The practice of martial arts extends far beyond the hands or balance. The mental aspect of this discipline is something that is one of its appeals to pros and amateurs. After he left the Cowboys, Inosanto sent Ward the following note and poem that he wrote:

Dear Bob,

Find your way and climb.

- Dan

"We are climbing different paths through the mountain of life
And we have all experienced much hardship and strife.
There are many paths through the mountain of life
And some climbs can be felt like the point of a knife.
Some paths are short and others are long
Who can say which path is right or wrong?
The beauty of truth is that each path has its own song
And if you listen closely you will find where you belong.
So climb your own path true and strong
But respect all other truths for your way for them could be wrong."

- DAN INOSANTO

• • • •

The building is a non-descript, gray warehouse in an industrial area east of downtown Dallas. This small building is the type of place you have to want to find to have any interest in being there. Inside the quaint structure is a boxing ring that nearly takes up the entire square footage of a workout facility that is humid, hot, and uncomfortable. Along the walls are famous boxing promotional posters as well as several karate and mixed martial arts pictures. Included in this array of décor is a photo of Bruce Lee and Dallas Cowboys Hall of Fame defensive tackle Randy White. This is the workout studio of Val Espiricueta (Es-pear-eeh-quet-ah). Val, who in 2015 was 57, remained in tremendous physical condition. Espiricueta is a personal trainer who teaches boxing and, primarily, martial arts.

"Bob was the first guy to do this," Espiricueta said. "People don't realize how useful and how valuable this can be to a player. The conditioning. The training. The balance. The hands. The speed. All of it is right there. I can't believe no one had seen this before Bob."

Espiricueta has trained players such as NFL Pro Bowlers DeMarcus Ware, Jay Ratliff, La'Roi Glover, Greg Ellis, Andre Gurode, as well as Ben Gardner, Tyrone Crawford, and countless other players. The benefits for the NFL players are one specific area – hand work. If an NFL player believes it works, he will pay the high price required to train with Espiricueta. When applied properly, the techniques taught by Espiricueta can be highly beneficial.

"When [former Dallas Cowboys Pro Bowl defensive end] Greg Ellis came to me, we had worked out for years. He was the one who introduced me to DeMarcus Ware, but he didn't do it until the final year or so of his career," Espiricueta said.

Ellis wanted to keep his job and remain important to the Cowboys. He didn't want to give Ware, who would eventually become of the NFL's most dynamic pass rushers in his era, any reason to be any better than he already was. Ware's speed was superior to most people he faced. Ware would become a consistent client of Espiricueta's.

"If I didn't learn martial arts, I'd be just a basic dip-and-rip guy just trying to go around the corner," DeMarcus Ware said. (Dip-and-rip is a football term defensive players use to describe how a player drops their shoulder and uses their arm to move past or around a blocking offensive player).

Greg Ellis had warned Ware, "You are not going to have this speed forever, but you can have the quickness."

The martial arts movements can be especially brutal and frustrating when applied properly. When the Dallas Cowboys played the Tennessee Titans on Oct. 1, 2006, Cowboys center Andre Gurode was especially effective against one of the most dominant defensive lineman in the NFL, Titans' tackle Albert Haynesworth.

"He was mad because Andre was kicking his ass," then Dallas Cowboys quarterback Drew Bledsoe said.

After one particular play, Gurode's helmet had come off as he was thrown to his back on the field. Haynesworth was so mad and frustrated that he deliberately stomped on Gurode's exposed head and narrowly missed causing more damage to his face than he already did. Haynesworth was ejected from the game, fined $190,000, and suspended an unprecedented five games by the NFL.

"It changed the whole system of playing. [Martial arts] in football is different. It is weird," Espircueta said. "People are not used to doing it, especially for football. Bob Ward was doing the same thing. He was trying to teach a system of martial arts."

Former Stanford University defensive lineman Ben Gardner, who was drafted by the Dallas Cowboys in 2014, quickly became a believer in the power of martial arts in football. Gardner was a seventh round draft pick and was looking for any advantage.

"I developed two completely new moves, but the more pivotal part is developing the instincts to do [them] naturally where you don't even think about it," Gardner said. "To be able to get other people's hands off of you without even thinking about it. It is a little unconventional – most football players think, 'It's the offseason, I have to get stronger and stronger.' The crux of line play in football is hand play and hand violence, and I do think more people would benefit from it."

More and more players do, but it's not called martial arts or Wing Chun. Today, it's called Ultimate Fighting.

• • • •

The inception, growth, and immersion of Mixed Martial Arts (MMA) has attracted NFL players to the sport as viewers and amateur participants. MMA is more commonly referred to as Ultimate Fighting Championship; it is a combination of boxing, wrestling, and martial arts. Its combatants do not wear any protection and fight in an octagon-style ring in rounds lasting five minutes. It can be a bloody spectacle, and it is wildly popular.

Fox Sports NFL reporter Jay Glazer, along with former MMA fighter Randy Couture, successfully built a small brand of training NFL players in MMA fighting. These relationships have also made Glazer one of the most successful NFL media "insiders" – reporters who are full of private information – in sports journalism today. Among some of his higher profile clients are NFL players Keith Rivers, Patrick Willis, Ryan Grant, Matt Leinart, and Jared Allen. It is worth noting that in today's era of NFL players, and more specifically NFL contracts, many defensive players have incentives in their deals stipulating certain benchmarks, i.e. if a guy records so many sacks, he receives a bonus of $100,000. There is financial incentive to train this way.

Glazer used mostly Muay Thai experts for his training with an emphasis in balance and leg drive. It is similar to what Ward was doing with the Cowboys in the '70s. In May of 2010, Glazer told *The New York Times*, "We want to revolutionize athletic training."

This particular athletic training revolution had already happened on the practice fields in Thousand Oaks, California when Bob Ward first introduced Dan Inosanto to the Dallas Cowboys.

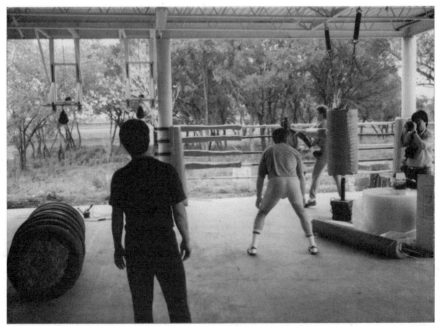

Bob Ward designed and had installed a half boxing ring at the Dallas Cowboys' training facility in 1985 at Valley Ranch. The ropes had springs that were energy producers for maximum repetitions.

CHAPTER **11**

PERFORMANCE ENHANCERS: THE GOOD, THE ABUSED, & THE ILLEGAL

"The continued search for a 'Magic Charm' or 'Drug'
that can transform a man into a hero is a myth deeply
ingrained in the human spirit, and can only be dispelled
by persuasion founded on scientific evidence."
– G. J. La Cava

Bob Ward tried steroids in the '60s. They were legal, and he figured he would try 'roids based on what he'd read in medical journals and the benefits he saw to the world-class athletes he knew. He wanted to see for himself if they worked; if they would change his body structure, increase muscle mass, and improve his distance throwing and how much weight he could lift.

The "testing" and the results left zero doubt: Steroids did what they said they would do. As an avid weight lifter, amateur athlete, and mad scientist about athletic performance, he lived right in the middle of the steroid phenomena in the '60s and '70s. There was no way he was going to miss this trend or the potential to be bigger, faster, and considerably stronger. As a man who frequented Muscle Beach from its inception as a place where gymnasts performed acrobatic feats, to its current status as a premier destination for body builders, there was no way he could miss out on the "growth spurt" that was the world of anabolic steroids.

It wasn't hard since they weren't yet illegal. He bought Dianabol and used it for two cycles in the mid-'60s while he was coaching at Fullerton Community College. What he experienced was the same thing that everybody else who ever took steroids did – they worked.

Steroid use is a complicated issue for Bob Ward. Considering his timeline as an athlete and coach, he falls right in the direct ascension of the study and proliferation of steroid use. He experienced their benefit and, peripherally, their potential destruction; he also witnessed how attitudes toward their use dramatically shifted during his professional career.

Steroid use was easily the most tawdry, marketable, and noticeable supplement in the rapidly growing, constantly changing world of nutrition, vitamins, diet, and additives that Ward delved into during his career.

"Forget for a moment about steroids and just think about this – American football is roughly a $200 billion industry, and the dietary and supplement business is $6 billion a year," former Cowboys and Denver Broncos wide receiver Butch Johnson said. "Before that, we ate steak and lifted. The introduction of what you put into your body is not just about steroids. It's a massive global business that includes steroids and everything else, too."

In the '60s to the early '70s, when steroid use was in its infancy, no one had any clue as to the negative effects of steroids or that their use would eventually be deemed illegal, banned, and something that would stain sports and its users in future generations. But, back then, using steroids was akin to smoking cigarettes in the '30s and '40s – nobody knew better, so they did. And they did. And they did. And they did.

"I have no regrets about [using steroids] because, at the time, it was something new that came on the market, and we went to the doctor and did it under doctors' supervision," Hollywood icon Arnold Schwarzenegger said in an interview with ABC long after he'd won Mr. Universe in the '70s. "We were experimenting with it. It was a new thing. So you can't roll the clock back and say, 'Now I would change my mind on this.'"

Since the '70s, the additional means of performance enhancement have completely altered the way sports are played and viewed. In some cases, this portion of performance enhancement has tainted sports for multiple eras in multiple arenas. Just the term "performance enhancement" conjures images of cheating, but it is far more complex.

Performance enhancement is not solely about a syringe – it's about nutrients, the juggling act that is diet, hormones, water, and body weight.

• • • •

Ward says he never once gave any of his athletes at Fullerton Community College or the Dallas Cowboys steroids, and he never once told any of the athletes he trained at Fullerton or with the Cowboys where they could obtain steroids. If a player wanted to find out about steroids or where to get them, it wasn't hard – the Pittsburgh Steelers didn't get those huge arms from super nutrition alone. Ward said that many were well aware that players were using 'roids. But there was nothing he or virtually anyone else could do about it.

"You would see a guy come back after six weeks of being gone and he was 20 pounds bigger. You pretty much always knew when a guy was using them," he acknowledges.

Personally, Ward used steroids as a means to gain muscle mass and to improve recovery since one of the benefits of steroids is allowing muscles to recover far more quickly than they would if following a pattern of only rest. The fear Ward had was that anabolic steroids could help everything grow – including potentially dangerous cancerous cells. The fear of potentially fueling cancer cells was enough for him to stop using steroids, even if no doctor or researcher ever told him there was a link between the two.

He also sensed steroid use was going to become a major problem for sports and its advocates. Steroids, and more specifically being a lobbyist for their use, damaged his brother Paul's career.

When Bob Ward tried Dianabol – the steroid most widely used in the '60s – it was something the Soviets had explored and implemented in their Olympic athletic program.

"It had started earlier than the 1960s," USC All-American shot putter Dave Murphy said. "[U.S. Olympians] Randy Matson and Bob Hoffman were at the Opening Ceremonies of the 1964 Summer Olympics in Tokyo. Matson turned to Bob and asked, 'How many people here are using Dianabol?' Hoffman looked at him and said, 'Almost everyone here is using that.' It was widely used, and it was like everything else in that time period – it was abused."

The problem with steroids or any synthetic means of enhancement is, despite their side effects, they are often worth using. The chance to play, chance to be better, or the chance to earn more money make steroids nearly impossible to reject.

"Steroids weren't regulated, and you could pretty much do whatever you wanted," said former Dallas Cowboys offensive lineman Brian Baldinger, who played in the '80s. "I had guys that told me it was the difference between them making the team and making it in the NFL. It was prevalent in the NFL."

· · · ·

By the time Ward arrived to the Dallas Cowboys in 1976, there was one team that was always in their way for clear supremacy of the National Football League. Whatever the Dallas Cowboys did, the Pittsburgh Steelers did just a bit better. Beginning in 1974, the Steelers won four of the next six Super Bowls – two of which came at the expense of the Dallas Cowboys. Ask members of the Cowboys teams in the '70s, and many are convinced they were not quite as good as the Steelers *because* of steroids. For years, it was widely assumed that the Steelers were the pioneers of steroid use in the NFL, which was later validated.

"It started, really, in Pittsburgh," former Steelers player and NFL head coach Jim Haslett said in an interview in 2005. "They got an advantage on a lot of football teams. They were so much stronger [in the] '70s, late '70s, early '80s. They're the ones who kind of started it."

Steelers legendary owner Dan Rooney later challenged Haslett's words, but the latter did not back down from his statement. Haslett added later, "It's naïve to think people weren't using enhancing drugs before they were illegal."

It did not help Rooney's case that, in 1985, *Sports Illustrated* ran a story about retired Steelers offensive lineman Steve Courson, who told the magazine that 75 percent of the Steelers offensive linemen in the late '70s used steroids. His 1991 book, *False Glory: The Steve Courson Story*, alleged that steroid use was common in the NFL.

This does not mean every player from the Dallas Cowboys was an angel who avoided steroids. The Steelers weren't alone.

And it wasn't as if the Steelers were considerably bigger than every other team, including the Cowboys. Ward said he knew guys used them. The average weight of the Steelers' five starting offensive linemen in the 1978 Super Bowl was 253.4 lbs; the Cowboys' group was 252.8 lbs. The front seven defensive players – the bigger guys – for the Steelers combined to weigh 240.3 lbs. while the Cowboys were 244.6 lbs.

In the late '70s, the United States government had yet to ban their use. There was no reason for the NFL to test; public awareness on the issue was still low, and it was relevant in sports only every four years during an Olympic competition. The potential dangers were mostly silent. There was more reason for the NFL players to use than not. Ward had no way to patrol their use even if he wanted to.

As players got bigger, faster, stronger, and recovered more quickly, one of the reported side effects to steroid use is heightened aggression. Today, it's known as 'roid rage.

Cowboys president Tex Schramm asked Ward once in the early '80s if he thought it was a good idea for the team to give players steroids. Ward said no. Not because they didn't work, but because he sensed public sentiment would soon grow wary of the advisability of their use.

In 1990, after he left the Cowboys, Schramm was hired to be the president of the start up World Football League. Its offices were in the Dallas suburb of Las Colinas, and he invited Ward, who by then had left the Cowboys, to come by for a chat/interview.

"What do you think about steroid use?" Schramm asked Ward.

"I do believe it could have a place if done properly and under the proper medical supervision," Ward said.

Even today, Ward says, "All you have to do is look how 'hormone therapy' is used in the medical community to validate that it has a positive place in treating various hormone issues."

Ward remains firm on that stance regarding the use of steroids. "How can I refute that?" he asks rhetorically. "They work. I am not a medical doctor, and therefore, anything I've said is only my opinion based on the medical literature. Let's have the medical experts make the decisions on when to prescribe hormone replacement, or enhancements."

• • • •

There is some evidence that in original ancient Olympic Games, participants experimented with performance enhancing drugs, but the gold medal winner in terms of steroid-aided improvement belongs to the Soviet Union. The Soviets are hailed as the ones who first began to aggressively experiment, test, and implement steroids back in the '60s. A nod goes to the Nazis as well in this development; Adolf Hitler's band of cruel zealots tested a variety of drugs on its prisoners in the '40s during the Third Reich. The Nazis were renowned for human testing; despite the inhumane brutality of that practice, the results eventually leaked out to various researchers and scientists who took their findings and applied it forward long after the Nazis were defeated.

The Soviets and the East Germans are usually credited as the first leaders in research and implementation of steroid use in sports.

In 1928, the International Association of Athletics Federation became the first governing body for sports to ban the use of "doping" by its athletes. It was not until 1967 did the International Olympic Committee create a medical commission, and in 1968 the IOC began testing for "banned substances" both at the Winter and Summer Olympics; testing had not been developed to detect the use of anabolic steroids. That was the year both the first Olympian was disqualified for doping and the first time a horse would be DQ'd from the Kentucky Derby for using a banned substance.

After the fall of Communism, the opening of the East German secret police – the Staasi – documents revealed that more than 10,000 athletes were often unknowingly subjected to steroid use by their coaches and trainers. For more than a decade, the East German swim team dominated international competition, but their participants often paid a steep price for rampant steroid abuse; many reportedly suffered psychological problems and several delivered children that suffered from birth defects from the after-effects of drug use.

All the while, the NFL was sitting right there and had no policy about any such measures against steroid use. And NFL players had begun to dip their toe into drugs to see if they worked.

At that time, the most casual and common widespread drugs used were stimulants called amphetamines. They help keep a person awake, but have no correlation to speed, quickness, or strength. In the '70s, the use of cocaine started to become increasingly popular despite it already being illegal.

In 1973, three years before Ward was hired by the Cowboys, the head coach and the general manager of the San Diego Chargers, Harland Svare, was fined by the NFL after it came out that his team was using amphetamines. Coincidentally, when Ward was trying out for the New York Giants, Svare was a member of the team. Ward recalls seeing several players popping some amphetamines before a preseason game against the Green Bay Packers.

The public reaction to this news was so harsh the Chargers built an awning over the team's tunnel at the home stadium to prevent fans from throwing objects at Svare.

The outcry was so intense that Svare quit with six games remaining in the season. It did not help that the Chargers were 1-6-1 when he decided to quit. The swift reaction against Svare was such that players knew to be discreet about whatever it was they were taking. The use of anabolic steroids grew quietly nonetheless.

"It was off the books, but you knew about it peripherally that's for sure," said Cowboys safety Cliff Harris, who played for the team in the '70s. "I never used them, but both of my sons played college football and they would tell me you would not believe how much steroid use there was in college football. For me, I never wanted any part of it, but I didn't play a position where a guy like me would have wanted to use it."

• • • •

The NFL did not officially ban steroid use until 1983, which stopped approximately no one. Kevin Callaway was an offensive lineman who came to Cowboys training camp in 1984. He was a rookie free agent and a long shot to make the team.

"I do remember there was a point when I said something about steroids because they were giving me this herbal stuff. It wasn't Dianabol, it was just herbal," Callaway said. "One time, before I got to the Cowboys, I had tried Dianabol. I used them for three weeks. I was paranoid, and I thought, 'This is crazy.'"

Callaway recalls one day when he saw a player who came to training camp and, "You could see in his eyes he was wired. He was doing something," Callaway said. "I had knocked him on his butt during practice. He got up and he cold cocked me. [Quarterback] Danny White came up to me and said, 'Why did you let him do that?' I didn't let him do it; he came out of nowhere. It was a light bulb moment for me; sometimes, the best athletes are chosen, but sometimes, it's the guy who is using [steroids]."

By this time, the dirty secret about the NFL was steroid use. Guys were doing it, but it was more of a "don't ask-don't tell" policy. "In all my years, I never saw a guy actually take it," former Cowboys assistant coach Gene Stallings said.

"You heard guys talk about steroids, but it really was something you just never saw," former Cowboys defensive tackle Randy White said.

By the '80s, the use of anabolic steroids had evolved out of the Olympics and unofficially into the NFL and NCAA football. The players who were using them to get bigger and stronger were nearly all linemen or linebackers. The scientific advances made by the Eastern Europeans – specifically the Soviet Union and the Bulgarian weightlifting program – were now being perfected by American doctors and making a tremendous impact on the highest levels of football.

But studies were beginning to show that there were serious side effects to steroid usage, which in turn soured the ticket-buying public.

Before he became the conditioning coach of the Houston Astros, Dr. Gene Coleman was doing research studies for his graduate degree at the University of Texas in the early '70s. One of his colleagues was conducting research on the effects of steroids on players and "The problem was the law would only allow him to administer a pharmacological dose," Coleman said. "Meaning, he was allowed to replace with a synthetic what his body would normally produce."

The findings of such a test were negligible. As a result, the medical community looked at such research and dismissed steroids as mostly ineffective drugs.

"Well, then we would look at a guy who was clearly taking steroids and ask, 'Do you really think it doesn't work?'" Coleman said. "To test with a pharmacological dose said nothing. You had to test what the guys taking them were doing – three and four or five times the allowed dose. That's when you started to see the effects.

"It really was – 'Take something and throw it against the wall and see what happens.' The more you take, the better you get until it literally kills you. They didn't know any different. While steroid use wasn't in baseball then, nobody knew that those players were having a good time with Greenies [another term for amphetamines]."

The NFL didn't begin testing for steroid use until 1987. That was just about the time Bob Ward received some visitors from the NFL league office.

"The league had really started to try to get a handle on steroid use then and it sent a bunch of investigators and administrators to our offices at Valley Ranch," Ward remembers. "What they were doing was looking for something that was under the rug. They were fishing for anything they could find."

The NFL was looking for any recorded use of steroids. When it came to the Cowboys, there was nothing to find. When it came to the original crackdown on steroid users in the NFL, only a few flunked the test, yet their use was still prevalent. And few people within the respective team offices would have been dumb enough to maintain a recorded list of their distribution and any possible usage.

"For legitimate reasons, they didn't want any of that stuff around," Ward says. "I am sure some of our guys were taking it, but I had no part in any of it."

Players were getting bigger and bigger and bigger, and by the mid-to-late '80s, studies showed there were damaging side effects to their use and abuse. The abuse of anabolic steroids would likely result in high blood cholesterol levels, severe acne, baldness, fluid retention, high blood pressure, liver disorders, as well as birth defects and sexual and reproductive disorders.

As the use of anabolic steroid testing grew popular, so too did human growth hormone (HGH). Unlike steroids, which are clearly detectable in testing, HGH requires a far more advanced and expensive method to catch users.

Former Los Angeles Raiders and Denver Broncos defensive end Lyle Alzado died in 1992, seven years after his 15-year NFL career ended. He died of a brain lymphoma, a rare form of cancer, at the age of 43. In the latter stages of his life, he revealed he had abused steroids and HGH throughout his football career, from college to the NFL. Although doctors said there was no link between steroids and his cancer, Alzado was convinced he was dying because he abused those drugs.

It was that type of thinking – that steroids or HGH could expand and multiply any cells, including cancer – that alerted Ward to the dangers of their use in the mid-'60s.

• • • •

In the '70s, Bob Ward had seen enough to know that not only did steroids work, but their usage and their users were going to come under intense scrutiny. All you had to do was watch the Olympics to see this was going to be a problem. If something was associated with the Soviet Union, it was not going to go over well with the American public. There were those, however, who passionately defended steroid use and lobbied for their usage. Those who took such a stance paid a price, and Ward had to look no further for proof than his younger brother, Paul Ward.

Because exercise science apparently runs in the family, Paul Ward earned his PED from Indiana University and played football at Whitworth College, while the youngest Ward brother, Maury, did his Master's Thesis on steroid use when he was at Chapman University near Los Angeles.

For a brief period, Bob and Paul were at Indiana University together studying for their respective doctorates in the field of Biomechanics and Measurement and Evaluation; at the time, the Ward brothers were two of the three men in the U.S. to have their PED in that field. They would often make the 2,100-mile drive together from Southern California to Bloomington, Indiana, in an old Volkswagen. The sight of these two big guys cramped into an old Volkswagen had to be only slightly amusing.

Bob and Paul were both exceptionally bright, innovative men who made significant impacts in performance enhancement. In 1972, Paul Ward's dissertation at Indiana University was studying the two techniques used to start a sprint – standing or crouching. He eventually applied his findings and some of his specific research methods to the Cowboys after his brother was hired.

Paul Ward had been lifting weights with his older brother Bob since the time he was about 10 years old. Unlike Bob Ward, Paul Ward made it for a little while as a professional football player. A lineman, he played two seasons for the Detroit Lions in 1961 and 1962. With the Lions, he and teammate Bob Whitlow began working out with weights after practice on Ward's recommendation. Another teammate, Joe Schmidt, joined them; in 1961, Schmidt had muscle transplant surgery and was introduced to weight training as a potential improvement in his rehabilitation process. At the time, invasive surgeries for players were seen as the end of a career.

"The stuff you see now with guys ripping up their knees or their shoulders – that would be it," Hall of Fame quarterback Roger Staubach said. "Back then, if a guy tore his ACL in his knee or tore his rotator cuff [in his shoulder] they never came back from it. Now they do all the time."

When Paul Ward lifted weights after practice with the Lions, a steadily increasing number of his teammates joined. It wasn't long before the number of players easily out-numbered the amount of equipment at the Lions' modest training facility in Cranbrook Educational Community in Bloomfield Hills, Michigan.

Joe Schmidt was a Pro Bowler that season, and one of the players who decided to join the post-practice weight room workouts was a cornerback named Dick LeBeau. LeBeau went on to enjoy one of the longest careers in professional football and was one of the top defensive coordinators in the history of the league; in 2015, he was still a defensive coordinator in the NFL, at the age of 77, and was inducted into the Pro Football Hall of Fame in 2010 for his career as a cornerback. The man has been in professional football for nearly 60 years.

In 1961, Paul Ward trained at the Sayer Park YMCA in Chicago, next to a man Clyde Emrich. Emrich was a U.S. Olympian who had competed in the 1952 Olympics and, in 1957, set the middle heavyweight world record in the clean and jerk. Emrich would be hired by Bears founder George Halas in 1971 as the team's strength coach, one of the first in the NFL.

During Paul Ward's tryout with the Bears, one of the men he trained with who made a deep impression on him was defensive end Doug Atkins. At 6-foot-8, 275 pounds, Atkins was one of the first "freaks" in the NFL. Atkins was so strong, he could throw opposing offensive linemen; Baltimore Colts guard Jim Parker admitted that after facing Atkins he nearly quit. Atkins played 17 NFL seasons and was a Pro Bowl selection eight times; he was inducted into the Pro Football Hall of Fame in 1982.

Exposure to men such as Atkins and Emrich made an enormous impact on Paul Ward, and eventually Bob Ward.

It was in the NFL, when steroids were still legal, that Paul Ward began to try what he said were "small amounts of" Dianabol. He later wrote a pair of studies on steroids and discovered that "10 milligrams of Dianabol produced significant increases in strength and lean body mass in athletes while training with weights over a relatively short period of time."

When Bob Ward accepted the job with the Cowboys, he invited Paul to come down and pick his brain about any ways he could think of to improve the team.

In 1982, Dr. Paul Ward was working with the United States Olympic Committee's Elite Athlete Project. He was a voluntary coordinator of a program for shot putters as well as discus, javelin, and hammer throwers. Ward caused a stir when, in 1984, he was quoted in a story in the *Los Angeles Times* stating that he had given some athletes in that program advice and information about how to beat drug tests for anabolic steroids. After that article appeared, the USOC cut ties with Dr. Paul Ward.

USOC executive director F. Don Miller said in a statement that "This man does not represent the vast majority of our athletes with his views on drugs and how to avoid detection of their use. He has done a tragic disservice, an injustice, to our goals for a drug-free amateur sports family by his widely publicized stance and activities."

The nobility of that statement was nice, but Dr. Paul Ward was far from the only man with the knowledge to beat a steroid test. Dr. Paul Ward was now viewed as an advocate for something that was beginning to be deemed dangerous and illegal by the government. A few days later, Dr. Paul Ward was granted space in the *Los Angeles Times* to write a rebuttal. He flatly denied ever advising athletes to use anabolic drugs, nor how to take them.

He wrote in the article for *The Los Angeles Times*:

"It is a fact, however, that many international athletes are using anabolic substances with impunity, yet are not found to be positive when tested. Drug usage among athletes is a serious problem, but testing has failed to curtail its use. The testing program simply increases the use of less detectable types of anabolic steroids and other new drugs. As a result of this ineffectiveness, the testing of athletes results in arbitrary, and thus unfair, enforcement of the drug ban. ... Amateur athletes are handicapped by the USOC's failure to implement alternative training, nutritional, and psychological programs that would eliminate the athletes' perceived need for drug usage. Drugs in sports will be a problem until the USOC deals with the reasons athletes take drugs and not just discovering that they do."

For the record, Dr. Paul Ward believes steroid use in limited doses administered by a professional has benefits and should be allowed with strict guidelines. "I believe that I provided the necessary science and research that demonstrated the correct usage that would not harm the athlete or average person if they used the lower form," he said. "In addition, if the person would use the low level while monitored by a doctor or trainer who is educated, that will demonstrate the effective results of the low level usage for athletes and body builders."

He remained in his executive position with Bally's Fitness until 1989.

• • • •

In 2015, every major sports league across the world has adopted steroid and HGH testing. But how much these measures have worked to combat or counter performance enhancing drug use is merely a guess. Despite increased testing and awareness, drug use in sports was rampant from the '90s through the current era. Performance enhancing drugs are no longer just for weight lifters, body builders, football players, or big guys.

Sports such as cycling, baseball, and running were all as affected by performance enhancing drug use like football had been years earlier. High profile athletes such as seven-time Tour de France champion Lance Armstrong and baseball's all-time home run leader Barry Bonds have been linked to steroid use. While fewer and fewer football players test positive for steroids any more, it's highly likely that the results are simply a matter of not being caught.

"You have started to see how tailored and well-masked [performance enhancing drugs] are with the highest level athletes and the greatest doctors working together to produce the best athletes money can buy," said veteran trainer Brian Weese who worked at Texas Tech and now prepares NFL hopefuls. "They figured out how to mask every possible marker. To this day, it still gets done. Don't think it doesn't. They figured out how to mask every marker that can come up in a test."

Steroids are currently permitted through prescription only, and there are a number of benefits beyond that to a football player or a baseball home run hitter. To sports researchers, the benefit of a steroid – in a limited dose – should be permitted; the thinking is that in a limited use, it can accelerate recovery. It would be akin to taking an aspirin – why wouldn't you take it if it worked?

That is Dr. Bob Ward's position – a steroid is a drug like any other that can help. If applied correctly, it should be permitted. However, he stresses that any drug should be done only with constant monitoring under a doctor's supervision.

"For one, I don't think the drug testing works," said Olympic gold medal middle distance runner Dr. Peter Snell. He competed in the Olympics in the

'60s, before he earned his PhD in Exercise Physiology from Washington State. He later went on to work at the University of Texas-Southwestern Medical Center in Dallas and conducted research with Bob Ward in the early '80s.

"The drug testing is expensive, too. Scientists are routinely developing ways to mask [performance enhancing drugs]. So, and this may be controversial, you allow a certain level. I am thinking more about EPO than testosterone."

EPO is erythropoietin, the drug mostly known as the performance enhancing drug of choice for Lance Armstrong during his run of Tour de France titles. "The rationale is, 'All I am doing is making my red blood cell count the same as someone else's,'" Snell said. "If it's controlled, the levels can be kept at a level which is safe rather than what is potentially to a point that could be very high and dangerous."

Snell's point is if a mature adult is making these decisions to do this to his body, it's on him. Snell is not an advocate for such usage for teenagers. For steroids to be accepted and allowed in any in sports, a societal shift will need to occur, similar to the current trend toward the legalization of marijuana.

Bob Ward was not a conduit or advocate of steroid use to the Dallas Cowboys, but he was a big believer in searching for other safe and healthy forms and alternatives of enhancing performance. He had to convince head coach Tom Landry that a water break was essential, so he instituted an "on field method" for providing players with an adequate supply of water during practice. The Cowboy trainers, headed by Don Cochren, managed the water system during practice. Ironically, studies show now that too much water is detrimental to athletic performance. In addition, current studies show that intelligent reduction of water causes the body to super-adapt and increase its ability to use water. This is clear evidence that constant research must be done to validate what coaches and athletes use to base their training decisions.

Ward provided Coach Landry with the scientific evidence so that he could provide adequate nutrition for the Cowboys' "training table" – the term most commonly associated with "food" for sports teams. Ward was a believer in the popular weight-gain powders that, by the mid-'70s, had become pretty much a constant at gyms across the U.S. If you wanted to get big, or bigger, and didn't want to take an anabolic steroid, "super nutrition" and supplementation including adequate protein, carbohydrates, fats, vitamins, minerals, water, and electrolytes was the way to go. Throughout his career and since he was a teenager, Ward searched for and took the scientifically supported nutrition of the day.

Ward certainly was not the first man to come to the NFL who was cognizant of the value or importance of what a player puts into his body as fuel, but he was certainly part of the movement that re-shaped how society viewed foods, herbs, and vitamins.

Today, it is not uncommon for trainers to stress to that people should eat every four to six hours. Sometimes more often. In the mid-'70s, when Ward arrived to the Cowboys, the three-meals-a-day routine was still widely practiced. Ward changed that by implementing cycles that were based on protein, carbohydrates, and fats that should be consumed every four to six hours, based on the hormonal activation in the human body.

He broke it down to snacks and regular meals in 1976. By 2015, most major fitness programs and training tables endorse similar patterns:

GAME DAY MENU
- Eat last meal prior to the game three to four hours before the start.
- Eat a small snack 30 to 45 minutes before the start of the game.
- Eat a small snack at halftime.
- Small snack after the game.
- Two hours after the game was the time to eat a larger meal.

Look at any food chart today that is designed for exercise and weight loss, and Ward was preaching the same diet in 1976 – it's all common sense: Omelet, cantaloupe, toast, tuna fish, orange, apple, steamed vegetables, sliced turkey, chicken breast, cottage cheese. Basically, if it's boring – go with it. These foods are the foundations for some of the most popular diets on the market, packaged, and sold for $24.99 on bookshelves today.

And the idea that all calories are the same – something that weight loss programs of this generation and diet books have stressed – is not correct. New research has clearly shown that one calorie is not the same as another; that a calorie generated by a Coca-Cola is not the same as a calorie generated by an apple.

In 2014, a documentary by former NBC and CBS news anchor Katie Couric titled *Fed Up* covered the growing epidemic of obesity in the United

States; Dr. David Ludwig, the director of the obesity program at Boston Children's Hospital, argued that calories generated from foods such as beans, nuts, and non-starchy foods such as vegetables are different than those from foods such as sugar, bread, and potatoes (starch). Dr. Dariush Mozaffarian, an associate professor of medicine and epidemiology at Harvard, states in the film that science saying people grow fat based on calorie consumption is outdated.

• • • •

Performance enhancement is not all about 'roids and illegal drugs. Roids and performance enhancing drugs are the parts of performance enhancement that receive the most attention because they're considered cheating and create headlines that often expose yesterday's winner as tomorrow's loser.

In the purest sense, performance enhancement is just about food, vitamins, dietary supplements, protein powder, sleep, rest, when you should eat, and an assortment of less tawdry elements that don't sell newspapers but actually do work.

Ward's Words
Stealing from the Steelers

Every team in the National Football League tried to, or did, copy the Dallas Cowboys thinking they were going to be as good as we were. There was only one team that was as good as we were, so naturally there was one area where we tried to copy them. I was like everybody else with the Dallas Cowboys in the '70s – We planned and worked hard to beat the Pittsburgh Steelers for no other reason than they beat us. The Steelers won four Super Bowls in the '70s, two of which came against the Cowboys; I was with the team when we lost the Super Bowl in 1978. I have never seen a game with more talent.

The Steelers were entirely about intimidation, which when done right, can be achieved through nothing more than appearance. As history told us later, the Steelers of the '70s were one of the NFL teams that were pioneers in the use of anabolic steroids. At the time, it was not a widely known fact. What was widely known was that they were big, and they looked intimidating. The Steelers, especially their offensive and defensive linemen, all featured big, muscular biceps. Biceps are the guns, they are the flash. As an actual practical muscle for a football player, they don't do much; give me a football player with a strong mid section over the guy with the big biceps any day.

One day after the '78 season, we were in a coaches' meeting and one of the guys said our players need big biceps like the Steelers. Was the reason we lost two Super Bowls to the Steelers because of biceps? No. But I have always been a believer in you try everything to find what works. If a player believes big biceps are the reason they are having success, then that is the reason they are having success. I also knew that big biceps can potentially create the illusion of a physical mismatch between players because guys with big biceps look intimidating.

I knew the reality, but I was excited about doing this. I knew it would motivate guys to work out. I specifically designed a program to enlarge our players' biceps; whoever had the biggest flexed bicep at the end of training camp would be awarded a "championship belt." I also had other incentives like days off and the use of a car at training camp.

The guys were into it, and immediately, players like Randy White, Tom Rafferty, and countless others started doing more curls, pull-ups, and other exercises to get their guns loaded.

One day, wide receiver Butch Johnson came to me because he wanted his biceps bigger, too. As a wide receiver, he was never going to win this belt, but he wanted in on the fun. He wanted to look good in a tight shirt. I set up the weight racks, and bam-bam-bam *we raced through a hard workout to get those biceps pumped. It wasn't a disaster, but close; the next day, Butch's arms were so over-worked and over-taxed by the workout, he suffered what is known as "rhabdomyolysis" – it's a breakdown of the muscle tissue that leads to the release of muscle fiber contents into the blood. He couldn't extend his arms, and he was sore for days.*

Butch didn't win the award; that distinction went to defensive tackle Randy White, who was already the strongest player on the team. He was able to expand his biceps to 19 inches.

We didn't win the Super Bowl the next season, and after Randy White won the Biggest Biceps championship belt, the coaches who were so adamant about our guys having "bigger guns" were now on to the next thing.

CHAPTER 12

THE EMPIRE CRASHES

"Before something great happens, everything falls apart.
– Unknown

Bob Ward was already in the coaches' locker room at the team's headquarters in Dallas when Tom Landry walked in. It was the rare instance when the two men were alone in the same place. It was 1984, and for the first time since the early days of the Landry regime, it seemed that the Cowboys were no longer *the* Cowboys – Texas Stadium was no longer a guaranteed sellout and the team had not been to the Super Bowl since 1978.

The local media and the local fan base had begun to tire of not winning Super Bowls and not winning the way this franchise did for the better part of a decade. There was a man on this coaching staff – offensive coordinator Paul Hackett – who was rumored to be the heir to replace Landry, whenever he decided to retire. Landry had been in the same job since the Cowboys' inception in 1960.

Inside the coaches' locker room, Landry and Ward exchanged some banal small talk before the head coach said, "I'm about ready to turn this over to the younger guys, and they can take over. I'm getting too old to do this."

What does one say when Tom Landry says he is thinking about quitting as head coach of the Dallas Cowboys? Ward reacted nervously, in disbelief that his boss would make such a stunning revelation. "Oh, Coach, you don't mean that," Ward carefully responded, "Don't give up. You got a lot left in you."

That ended the exchange since more coaches began filing into the locker room to dress for another practice. Ward thought that Landry was actually going to retire.

• • • •

When the '80s began, there was no sign that the dominance of the Dallas Cowboys was going to change, despite the retirement of Roger Staubach. From 1980 to 1982, the Cowboys reached three consecutive NFC title games with Danny White as quarterback. They were the road team and lost all three, but there was one particular game that signaled the unofficial end of the Cowboys' definitive place at the top of the NFL.

On January 10, 1982, Ward took his customary spot in the coaches' box at Candlestick Park to watch the Cowboys play the San Francisco 49ers, who were then coached by Bill Walsh and quarterbacked by a blonde kid from Notre Dame named Joe Montana. According to Las Vegas oddsmakers, the Cowboys were three-point favorites to win this, the NFC title game and the right to go to the Super Bowl.

The Cowboys took a 27-21 lead in the fourth quarter. With a little less than five minutes remaining in the game, the 49ers had the ball 89 yards away from a go-ahead touchdown. Montana led the 49ers on a 14-play drive that ended with one of the most famous plays in NFL history. The

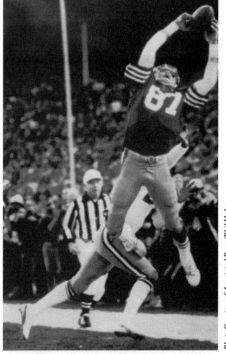

Photo Courtesy of Associated Press/Phil Huber

49ers had the ball six yards from a touchdown with 58 seconds. On the famous third-down play, Montana drifted to his right and lofted a pass that was intended to go out of bounds, but tight end Dwight Clark made a spectacular leaping catch in the corner of the end zone right over Cowboys cornerback Everson Walls for the play that would define a decade.

It is now simply referred to as "The Catch."

Sitting in the coaches' box, Ward couldn't believe what he saw and had no idea what this moment would mean. He knew sports, and life, is ultimately determined by a fingertip, by 36 inches. Both teams had trained for this moment, but in that fraction of a second, one guy simply made a play.

"The Catch" – San Francisco 49ers tight end Dwight Clark soars above Dallas Cowboys cornerback Everson Walls to catch then 49ers quarterback Joe Montana's pass to tie the NFC title. The 49ers went on to win Super Bowl XVI, the first of five Super Bowl victories in 14 seasons.

These were the plays the Cowboys had previously made, and now it was Montana-to-Clark. The Cowboys still had a chance to win the game, but after "The Catch," Cowboys wide receiver Drew Pearson caught a ball and a 49ers defender used a horse collar to prevent what would have been a potentially big play that would have helped the Cowboys re-take the lead. Alas, it was San Francisco's time. The 49ers won the game by one point. The Cowboys would be replaced by the 49ers, and Landry/ Staubach would be effectively succeeded by Walsh/Montana. The 49ers would become the NFL's team of the '80s with four Super Bowl wins.

The following season saw a nasty players' strike from NFL players that lasted 57 days and reduced the regular-season schedule from 16 games to nine. Although the playoffs were a tournament, the Cowboys did reach another NFC title game. They lost to rival Washington and would not reach the title game again until the 1995 season.

It was over only nobody, including Ward, knew it.

• • • •

More changes began to come in 1984 when the team's original owner, Clint Murchison, sold the Dallas Cowboys to an oil and gas businessman named H.R. Bum Bright. Bum wasn't a bad owner, but he wasn't a hands-off owner like Murchison had been. But, at that point, it may not have mattered who was signing the checks for the Dallas Cowboys – they simply weren't quite as good as some of the other teams in the NFL.

For the next few seasons, the Cowboys were still a good team, but they were no longer the premier team that they had been. Ward was still doing his job the way he had since he arrived in 1976, and exercise science, along with the specifics about his job, was well on its way to becoming the global industry it has become.

Thanks largely to Bob Ward, for a few years, the Cowboys were indeed ahead of nearly every other team in terms of fitness. By the mid-'80s, that was no longer the case. Specifically, the Eastern European methods that much of Ward's practices were rooted in had begun to change, too. Ward's willingness to share information played a role in this as well – something that would never happen today. In today's era of the NFL, to openly share is to die.

The scientist part of Ward's brain may have cost him and the Cowboys. Beginning when he was hired in 1976 and for the better part of a decade,

Ward exercised a near open door policy to his research and testing. That's what scientists do – they share information in the name of finding solutions and answers. Scientists, not coaches in an ever-increasingly competitive league.

In 1986, near the offices of the Dallas Cowboys, Ward held a "Sports Speed" Symposium that featured a who's who of sports strength, sports science, and sports conditioning experts. There were representatives from the NHL, the University of Wisconsin, the Digital Equipment Company, the University of Georgia, Stanford, the New York Jets, the University of Florida, the San Diego Chargers, Washington State, and on and on. The noticeable absentees from the conference were representatives from teams from the NBA and MLB; the respective leagues and sports were about a decade away from embracing strength training the way it exists today.

Dr. Jim Counsilman, who coached the USA swimming team during the Summer Olympics in 1964 and 1976 attended the event, too; during his time as the head coach of the swimming and diving program at Indiana University, his team won six consecutive NCAA titles. After the conference, Counsilman said, "This was the best symposium I've ever attended."

The event was great, but that it was led by a man from a prominent NFL franchise who was unknowingly giving away "trade secrets" was not so wonderful. By the early to mid-'80s, as the money in the league began to rise, so did the paranoia.

In 1986, team president Tex Schramm told Ward in no uncertain terms, "No more research!"

Even Tom Landry once said to Ward, "Bob, you let too many people in."

They weren't blaming their strength and conditioning visionary, but the collective strain of losing after so much winning was finally taking its toll. Tempers were shorter. Egos were bruised. Hubris had its way.

All of the innovation, technology, and organization that had put the Cowboys so far ahead for so long there was no longer an advantage. Nearly every other team was doing everything they had been doing, too. And, in many cases, they were doing it better.

"Once they started really sharing all of that information, they lost that edge," former Cowboys fullback Timmy Newsome said. "They were still attempting to take chances, but everybody had the same information. That is what cost the Cowboys."

In today's NFL, sharing is now associated with professional suicide. Open door policies are non-existent. Practices are open for the briefest of periods to only the media that covers the team – during the season, the standard time to watch is about 10 to 15 minutes.

The list of people Bob Ward invited to join him at the team's facility either in Dallas or at the new building in Valley Ranch was extensive. There is no doubt his findings impacted other trainers, coaches, doctors, and researchers.

Around that time, men such as Boyd Epley at the University of Nebraska under head football coach Tom Osborne had indirectly taken the origins of Ward's workouts and "Americanized" them. The diffusion of Ward's methods, or those emerging from the same philosophies, had a definite impact how athletes trained.

"More and more teams were drafting bigger guys and making them bigger," former Cowboys, Indianapolis Colts, and Philadelphia Eagles offensive lineman Brian Baldinger said.

Offensive and defensive lines were going big; in this case, bigger was not just better but essential. Under head coach Joe Gibbs, the offensive line of the Washington Redskins was nicknamed "The Hogs." While steroids were now banned in the NFL, dietary supplements and other means of adding muscle mass and bulk had become the rage in the league. And players were still using steroids, too – they just weren't getting caught.

Or they were.

Although steroid use was deemed illegal, usage was rampant. In 1985, the strength coaches at the University of Vanderbilt and Auburn University were both found guilty of trafficking steroids. In 1986, the Department of Justice indicted steroid dealers in Florida and Texas, and eventually, that same investigation resulted in arrests in California, Illinois, and New Jersey. That same year, 25 players, including All-Americans Brian Bosworth of Oklahoma and Jeff Bregel of USC, were suspended from playing in college bowl games after they tested positive for steroids. That following spring, Cowboys first-round draft pick Danny Noonan, who played at Nebraska, told scouts he used steroids to prepare for the NFL Combine.

The league was changing, growing, and so were the players. The Cowboys were not changing with it. Some of that reluctance to change can be explained by the lure of routine, by arrogance, by age, or fatigue.

One particular exchange eventually found its way into the 1990 book *God's Coach: The Hymns, Hype and Hypocrisy of Tom Landry's Cowboys*, written by Skip Bayless, long-time writer for *The Dallas Morning News*. The book was written to not humanize but to demonize Landry and expose him as a militaristic coach unworthy of the worship he'd received for nearly 20 years. Basically, the book was intended to portray America's Team as just another team doing business in order to shock readers and, of course, sell more books.

In the book, Bayless quotes Ward in a seemingly off-the-cuff training camp conversation where Ward tells of a time one late afternoon where he was sharing some data he'd compiled with Tom Landry when he noticed Coach was nodding off. Ward wasn't sure what to do, so he just kept on talking. He'd off-handedly mentioned it to Bayless, really as much as a self-deprecating indictment of his own complicated, maybe even tedious, compilation of data as it was a humorous anecdote and fond memory of Landry.

Bayless used the scene to paint the portrait of an older man who was so beyond "with it" that he couldn't stay awake at work. Ward regrets supplying any type of material that could be misconstrued as a criticism of a man he so revered – Landry.

• • • •

Unbeknownst to both Ward and Landry, the mid-to-late '80s was the finale of their time together with the Cowboys. Neither of them had any idea that the end would come in the form of a brash Arkansas billionaire who had dreamed of owning and running a professional football team for more than two decades.

Landry was indeed in the final stages of a brilliant career. He had built a team that posted 20 consecutive winning seasons, an NFL record. In that run, the Cowboys won 13 division titles, made the playoffs 18 times, went to the Super Bowl five times, and won twice. They had collectively revolutionized professional sports, and the Dallas Cowboys brand was synonymous with success.

What happened to the Dallas Cowboys happens to all empires, be it in sports, military, or government. Nothing lasts forever without a fall. What is so remarkable is not the way the fall occurred, but how long it took to actually happen and get ugly.

Beginning in 1984 and through 1988, the Cowboys made the playoffs one time and had two losing records. The one season they did make it – 1985 – they won 10 games, the NFC East Division title, but lost their playoff game by the score of 20-0 to the Los Angeles Rams. The Cowboys had overachieved for Landry's last winning season as head coach.

The Cowboys simply had set the bar too high for themselves and created a level of expectation that in an increasingly competitive NFL could not be sustained. Inevitably, it was all destined to end.

"There were a couple of things that precipitated it – the league caught up to their draft philosophy and the league had simply gotten bigger," Baldinger said. "The defense [the Cowboys] ran for so long under Ernie Stautner – the Flex – it no longer really worked as well. They had drafted better than anybody for years, and they had good quarterbacks. After Roger Staubach retired [in 1979], they had Danny White, and they were still good."

Even though White played under the foreboding cloud that Staubach would create for every single Dallas Cowboys quarterback, he was successful. The team had reached three consecutive NFC title games under White in the early '80s and remained competitive with him at quarterback. In the 1986 season, the Cowboys were 6-2 and had former University of Georgia and Heisman Trophy winning running back Herschel Walker in the same backfield with future Hall of Famer Tony Dorsett. The team also had a wide rookie wide receiver named Mike Sherrard, a first round pick from UCLA who, early on, was playing like a top player at his position.

"That was the most fun I ever had playing football in my career," Danny White said. "Defenses simply did not know what to do with Herschel Walker. We would come out of the huddle, and you could see they didn't know how to cover him. You could play him at any position. Playing quarterback had never been easier for me."

Entering the seventh game of the season, the Cowboys' offense was on pace to break a number of team records, and Danny White was en route to the most prolific statistical season of his life. In that seventh game, however, White suffered a broken wrist against the New York Giants.

"We completely fell apart when he went out," Baldinger said. "By that point in the NFL, if you didn't have a good quarterback, you were not going to have a very good team."

To put it lightly, the Cowboys were not a very good team without Danny White. They inserted Steve Pelleur in his place but were never the same. "It just completely changes the rhythm of a team when you change the quarterback," White said.

The team lost seven of their final eight games, and the following season they were 7-8 and missed the playoffs. Wide receiver Mike Sherrard, who looked to be the best Cowboys receiver since Bullet Bob Hayes or Drew Pearson, suffered a broken leg in 1987 training camp and never returned to the Cowboys. And defensively, they were simply inadequate.

"We just didn't have the talent that the other teams had," said defensive tackle Randy White, who would retire after the 1988 season. "You have to have talent."

This is the part of the equation that eventually gets everybody, especially a man such as Bob Ward. Coaches, analytics, research can all make you better, but eventually the ceiling is hit and the genetic code has been maxed out. If the guy across from you is working as hard with the same advances and has a higher ceiling and genetic code, that person will win. Always.

"We no longer had Roger, [linebacker] Lee Roy Jordan, Charlie Waters, Cliff Harris," White said. "When you look at why the Cowboys struggled or started to go down, it had to do with talent more than anything else."

Before the NFL put in a player salary cap in 1994, the primary methods of striving for parity among its franchises and to give each respective fan base the chance at having a winning team was the schedule and the Draft. The teams with the best records are annually slated with the most difficult schedules the following year; those same teams have the lower pick in the next spring's annual amateur draft.

For nearly 20 years, the Cowboys defied those mechanisms, thrived against the best schedules, and still found quality players despite the disadvantage of selecting lower in the draft. Those inherent obstacles simply never mattered, until they finally did. The harder schedules and the lower draft picks finally worked to expose a team that was simply no longer at the top.

"You keep drafting at the bottom, and it makes it so difficult. It is amazing they stayed where they did for as long as they did," said former Cowboys assistant coach Dan Reeves, who left the team in 1981 to take over as the head coach of the Denver Broncos. "They all did good jobs, but it was just a matter of time. All of those great players they had – Staubach, Randy White, Tony Dorsett – were all high draft picks. The odds are against you the lower you pick."

There were other components, notably a brain drain within the organization. It happens to every successful sports franchise – the top assistant coaches are hired by other teams.

Top Cowboys coaches like Dan Reeves, Mike Ditka, and Gene Stallings all left to take other head coaching positions. Reeves went to the Denver Broncos where, with Hall of Fame quarterback John Elway, he reached three Super Bowls. Ditka coached the Chicago Bears to the 1985 Super Bowl with what was the best defense in the modern era. Stallings went to the St. Louis Cardinals before he went to the University of Alabama where he led the Crimson Tide to a shocking win over heavily-favored Miami Hurricanes in the 1992 National Title game.

There was one other facet to this fall that Ward and others credit as a silent killer – the NFL Players Association strike. "There is no doubt that did hurt that team," said Cowboys safety Charlie Waters, who was not a part of the 1987 strike but had been a part of others. "We believed in fighting for the rights and for the guys coming after us, but those things do take a toll."

The NFL players' strike of 1982, which lasted 57 days, caused the NFL to eliminate seven regular season games. It also cost the players $275 million in lost revenues and wages, and the owners were forced to pay the networks that televised their games $50 million. These are complicated, stressful situations that put people who are on the same side directly across from the other; in this case, Danny White was attending meetings with Tex Schramm during the strike to discuss it.

"The longer the strike went on, the more I felt that this wasn't the players' strike, but [NFL Player's Union president] Ed Garvey's strike," Randy White told *The Dallas Morning News* in 1982. "All we did was waste eight weeks of football."

The Cowboys survived that strike to reach the NFC title game that season. When the players went on strike again, no team was hurt more than the Dallas Cowboys. "That really broke us up," Ward said. "It really tore that team apart."

One element to the Dallas Cowboys under Tex Schramm and Gil Brandt that is often under-played is how tough of contract negotiators they both were. They still operated in an era when owners and management could put the screws to players, which they routinely did. In 1987, the players went on strike, and in turn, the NFL responded by hiring replacement players. It was more commonly known as "scab football."

That meant Ward would come to work to train men who literally left their day job to pursue their dream of playing professional football. All of the coaches had no choice but to go to work, even though they knew it was essentially a waste of time. Players picketed, but this was a union that was fractured and no roster in the union was any more split than the Cowboys.

Established veteran Cowboys players such as Randy White and Tony Dorsett felt they had no choice but to cross the picket line and join a group of teammates who were teammates only in the sense they wore the same uniform. Schramm had negotiated contracts with both players that contained annuities that could be threatened if they didn't play. So, guys like Randy White and Dorsett played.

This put all of the coaches, especially Ward, in the inconvenient position of doing his job without appearing to be disloyal to the players who were on the other side of a fight he had nothing to do with. The problem for the coaches was the games counted in the standings – whenever the real players did return, the record would be impacted.

Ward didn't change what he did, and he recognized what it was for the temporary Cowboys: "For the guys off the street, it was a lifetime experience for them," he says.

The Cowboys were one of the better teams in the standings; in these "scab games," they finished 2-1. Their lone defeat in the replacement games came, ironically, at home with the likes of star regulars such as Danny White, Tony Dorsett, and Randy White playing a roster full of obscure Washington Redskins players. The Cowboys players, most notable Danny White and Dorsett, were openly booed at home by fans who did not want to hear players complaining about their six-figure salaries to play football. The Cowboys were eight-point favorites, but this game eventually became the inspiration for the 2000 Hollywood movie *The Replacements*, which starred Gene Hackman and Keanu Reeves.

The strike, overall, was fractured from the start. It lasted 24 days, cost three games off the schedule, and more than 10 percent of the NFL players crossed the picket line to play.

Despite the Cowboys' success in the standings during these replacement games, Ward is convinced this strike played a role in the destruction of the team. The Cowboys finished 7-8 that season, and it was readily apparent to those within and outside of the team that things were not going to improve the following season. Feelings were hurt, egos were bruised, and dissension was created between players, coaches, and management. Ward had nothing to do with that, but he was stuck dealing with it.

"I don't know about the one in 1987, but the one in 1981 was the one that really hurt us," Danny White said. "I think one of the biggest mistakes the Cowboys made, especially after the strike in 1981, was they didn't bring everybody together to patch things up. I know after the one in 1981, the San Francisco 49ers brought the whole team together, and they aired out their differences and they were a family again.

"I felt the wounds that were created by the strike in 1981 were never resolved for the Dallas Cowboys, and it did cause a problem."

The same can probably be said of the 1987 strike.

In 1988, the Cowboys finished a league worst 3-13 and very much earned the top pick in the NFL draft. Despite conversations between Tex Schramm and Tom Landry about the head coach possibly retiring, the latter stated after the season he planned to coach well into the '90s. As much as he is deified now, by the final two years of the Landry regime, some people wanted him out.

"People always forget that fans were screaming for Tom Landry to be fired. They said the game had passed him by," said the long-time voice of the Dallas Cowboys Brad Sham who, in 1988, also hosted a local radio sports talk show.

Ward knew changes would be made, but the change would be minor in light of the major overhaul that was coming.

• • • •

Bob Ward knew the Dallas Cowboys were for sale because he read about it in the papers. The reports circulating around the media was that Jerry Buss, the owner of the Los Angeles Lakers, would buy the Cowboys. Ward had been through the sale of the team before, but he had no idea how this was going to go down. Ward certainly had no clue that the man who would actually buy the team would become one of the most visible and influential owners in professional sports for the next quarter century.

On Feb. 24, 1989, Ward came home and told his wife that the coaching staff had just finished the best, most positive meeting they'd had in a long time. Coach Landry felt good about their prospects for the next season. Everyone was enthusiastic.

Ward was at work the next day when he heard the news: Team owner Bum Bright had sold the Dallas Cowboys and Texas Stadium for a then NFL-record $140 million. In 2015, according to *Forbes* magazine, the Dallas Cowboys are the most valuable team in the NFL worth approximately $4 billion.

That morning, Jerry Jones flew to Austin, Texas, to visit Tom Landry at his vacation home. He told Landry, "I'm here and so is Jimmy [Johnson]." He told Tom Landry he was fired. That evening at a press conference at the team's headquarters, Tex Schramm addressed a media gathering he had cultivated relationships with for more than two decades.

"It was a very difficult meeting," Schramm said during the press conference about meeting with Landry. "It's very, very sad. It's tough when you break a relationship you've had for 29 years. That's an awful long time."

Then-NFL commissioner Pete Rozelle told *The Dallas Morning News* that, "This is like Lombardi's death."

Jerry Jones said many years after, he wish he had waited one year to replace Landry; that he didn't know what he was doing in that first year, and that Landry could have potentially eased the transition. Buying the team meant Tex Schramm would leave shortly thereafter as well. It also meant the entire coaching staff would likely be replaced, too. Many front office employees were summarily fired as Jones made a complete overhaul of the organization to look the way he wanted. The job that Bob Ward had known since 1976, which had given him clout, fun, and a degree of celebrity was now very much in jeopardy.

That first evening, Ward went to visit Tex and asked him if he should contact former Cowboys assistants Dan Reeves or Mike Ditka about a job. Schramm told Ward not to resign just yet, to sit tight and to see what happened. Ward, who had one year remaining on his contract, agreed.

Jimmy Johnson did not fire Bob Ward, but he essentially demoted him. All of the powers, freedom, and responsibility Ward had under Tom Landry were gone. Clearly, Jimmy had a different vision for Ward's role and, more specifically, what he wanted from the players. It was, quite simply, a bad spot.

Ward immediately saw that the way Jimmy was doing things was not the way Landry had done them. Training camp under Jimmy was different. However, Landry was the only coach Ward had worked for in the NFL, so he had little to compare.

"We hit all the time," said Cowboys fullback Daryl "Moose" Johnston, who was a rookie that season. He played with the Cowboys until 1999 when a neck injury forced him to retire. "Jimmy's practices were absolutely brutal."

The first season under Jimmy Johnson, the team still trained in Southern California. The next year, they moved to St. Edward's University in Austin where Johnston said, "It was so much worse. I remember one time he was going to cut our water breaks because he thought we were drinking too much water. We were hitting twice a day. It was non-stop."

So much of what Ward had been allowed to do, even encouraged to do, from the research to the testing to the differing types of exercises was basically out. "Bob got put into a really hard spot to be in," Johnston said. "He was always upbeat and the most optimistic guy I've ever been around. But it was a hard situation to be in."

Ward had to do everything in his power just to encourage the new batch of players to workout at the team's facility. The weight room was covered with a roof, but it was not enclosed. Many of them preferred to go elsewhere in the area to workout.

"The job that I had was no longer the job I was hired to do," Ward reflects. "I had been so lucky to have that job, but Jimmy wanted his own guy to do things his way."

Ward was not one to openly complain, but he no longer enjoyed the job that he had previously loved. The team finished 1-15, and in shortly thereafter, Bob Ward told Jimmy to fire him.

"To have the career that I did with that team and to go out that way with that season was worse than *Dumb and Dumber*," Ward explains. "There was nothing I could do about it. I had just become a name there and a title to fill." Under any circumstances, it would have been difficult to walk away from that job – the highs, the respect, the glory, the notoriety, the money, and – of course – the players.

One morning, he came to work to box up his belongings and say goodbye to the many people with whom he'd spent countless hours over the previous years. So much of his professional life had been this team and with these people. And it was over. All of it. Ward would say publicly that he was relieved when he left the job, and in many ways he was, but it was still hard. This was a dramatic change to his life, so there would obviously be some separation anxiety. He was right at that awkward professional spot of being close to retirement age, but too young to not continue expanding his career.

Because the whole family had been involved in his time with the Cowboys, the change was emotional for all of them. He prayed often with his wife and family for some guidance in the direction he should take. He shed some tears when he thought about what could possibly replace the many highs associated with his work with this team. He still had aspirations in sports science.

"That was a really hard time for him," his oldest daughter, Shannon, said. "You have to remember, my dad had been always moving up his whole life. He was never still."

• • • •

Despite his vast experience, knowledge, and expertise in his field, Bob knew no NFL team would pursue him as a sports scientist, which was the direction he wanted to go. He wanted to apply all the knowledge he'd learned under Coach Landry's leadership in order to further improve the total football program quality in the NFL. At the time, though, other teams would be looking for the basic strength and conditioning coach, not a scientist. So, he made no attempts to find a new position in that particular coaching genre since, at that point in his career, he wasn't interested scaling back to what he saw was the beginning.

Instead, Ward joined with Dr. Ralph Mann to develop a business in "On-Field Analysis," the future of football analytics. They acquired NFL clients and analyzed their actual game performance for the coaching and scouting departments. Simultaneously, Ward worked for Dr. Phil Osborne in Shreveport, Louisiana, doing medical impairment evaluation.

Ward considered the possibility of returning to the academic world since he had truly loved coaching and teaching when he was at Fullerton, but after two inquiries back in his native California pointed out the difficulties he was likely to experience in pursuing that venue due to his over-qualification, he decided against making a move in that direction. With his doctorate and experience, and with the affirmative action and financing issues all meshing together, the likelihood of another dream job happening where he would want it to happen seemed improbable.

He eventually served as a consultant in martial arts for various NFL and college teams. By then, many teams had picked up on the martial arts idea and were already employing people in that capacity. The San Diego Chargers had him out to work with the linemen on martial arts training. He later applied for a similar job with the Cleveland Browns. The response letter from the Browns' head coach in 1993 read:

> "I, too, believe martial arts has a definite place in football programs today. In fact, the Cleveland Browns have been working with a local martial arts instructor, Joe Kim, for the past two years. So far, we have been extremely pleased with the results and intend to keep martial arts as a permanent part of our strength and conditioning program.
>
> Once again, Bob, many thanks for thinking of the Cleveland Browns.
>
> Sincerely,
>
> Bill Belichick
>
> Head Coach"

The real problem was that he was 57 and forever linked to a coaching staff that had been fired or, at the very least, deemed outdated. As a result, at least for the NFL, he was too old and his ways and methods were perceived as antiquated – even if they were far from it.

It would take more than 20 years before Dr. Bob Ward's profession would come around to fully validate that his way, more specifically his method of training, not only worked, but were the best. That his way made today's methods possible.

CHAPTER 13

FOOTPRINTS IN THE TURF

"Lives of great men all remind us, we can make our lives sublime, and, departing, leave behind us, footprints on the sands of time."
– *Henry Wadsworth Longfellow*

In the final month of the regular season of 1988, Bob Ward insisted to his family and friends that Tom Landry had a plan and that the demise of the Dallas Cowboys would be temporary. When the season ended, the team planned to select UCLA quarterback Troy Aikman with the first pick of the 1989 NFL draft. They already had wide receiver Michael Irvin. Both players would eventually join the Pro Football Hall of Fame.

Ward never got to see any of this through or even happen within the team. When he asked Jimmy Johnson to fire him – which was inevitable regardless of him asking – in the early months of 1990, it was an expected shock. Ward knew it was coming and was prepared for it, but not the surprise he felt. He was prepared to leave, but he would miss it. He would have liked to stay in the NFL, but his job role was not possible at that time.

His age and affiliation with an aging coaching staff essentially killed his chances at remaining in the league at a similar position with a different team. It did not help that a lot of people viewed Ward as an outlier and his job role completely impossible in the modern NFL.

"Guys like Bob Ward are threatening because people don't understand him," former San Francisco 49ers and Chicago Bulls strength and conditioning coach Al Vermeil said. "People are threatened by what they don't know, and he threatened people. What Bob Ward did to stay in Dallas for that long and to be that productive is incredible.

"If you want to find out about what kind of a coach he was or what people thought of him, talk to his players. Talk to the people he worked with and they all say the same thing."

And they do.

Ward never officially returned to the NFL, but years later, the NFL returned to Bob Ward to validate a career and a philosophy that was never truly outdated.

• • • •

In 1992, the year the Dallas Cowboys won the Super Bowl with Jimmy Johnson as the head coach and a full two years after Ward had been fired, a collection of the league's most prominent strength and conditioning coaches were interviewed for an article by *The New York Times*. The coaches offered the best exercises for football training, virtually all of which Ward was doing in 1976:

- Running with a parachute on your back. This resistance speed training was something Ward did with Danny White in the '70s.
- Running and sprinting hills. This is still regarded as one of the best forms of strength and cardiovascular work there is.
- Surgical tubing. This is what Ward had Charlie Waters do in 1977.
- Hand drills. This is what Ward introduced with martial arts expert Dan Inosanto.
- Repetitive motion. Now called "interval training," this is something Ward had the Cowboys doing in the '70s and '80s.

The New York Times article said, "The Cowboys lead the way," acknowledging the Cowboys as the leaders in strength training because, at the time, they were winning. "If the Cowboys had been winning in the last couple of years he was there, everybody would have been listening," Al Vermeil said. "It's monkey see, monkey do. Way too often guys in my position start winning and then they start bloviating how good they are and people believe them."

Ward is quietly convincing, but he is a horrible bloviator. The job that he had with the Cowboys did not exist elsewhere. He really was doing the job of two people, and no way would a personnel director want the input from a man in his position today. The level of paranoia that exists now in these jobs was foreign to Ward when he was in the league and has changed the mood around professional sports. "No one else would have given me the type of latitude and responsibilities I had," Ward recognizes. "It really was the perfect confluence of circumstances and timing. I was a conditioning coach by title, but really my specialty was personnel only for a guy with my background that job didn't exist."

One day, he was driving to the Cowboys' headquarters and caught himself thinking, "You've got it so good." He did, it just didn't last forever.

After he left the Cowboys, he went not into a depression but a rather deep funk. "That was a weird time for all of us," said his oldest daughter, Shannon. "He had never lost a job before. It just worked out that my husband and I moved from Oregon to Dallas around the time he left the Cowboys, and for a little while, I got a temporary job working [at a local church]. He would joke, 'You're the only one working.' We would laugh, but you knew that it was hard."

He tried for various jobs, including one in personal security; if someone paid him, he would have been a bodyguard. That never happened. "He would never let on, but you could tell he was frustrated," said his youngest daughter, Erin. "He would never yell, but you could tell he wasn't himself. I know he got turned down a lot."

The final portion of his professional career landed him at a pair of health-related companies, Mannatech and AdvoCare, for more than 15 years. Both companies sell themselves as "leaders" in the fields of sports research as well as health food and nutrition related products. At Mannatech, he was the director of Sports Science and Nutrition. He held a similar position at AdvoCare. There, he could do the type of sports and health-related research he wanted; it included studies conducted at the Indianapolis 500 as well as the Iditarod and with Olympic athletes. He aided in equipment design and delivered seminars that touched on his vast experiences.

Both of these places were good spots for Bob Ward to land; they certainly beat the alternative as a bodyguard for some high profile teen pop star or maybe teaching at a low-level college to a bunch of marginally interested students. These positions allowed him to remain a scientist, which, at his core, was what he'd been all along.

• • • •

Leaving the Cowboys and all the travel that involved gave Ward the chance to do something so many single-bread winning dads of his generation simply did not have the time to do – be around the house. But he was never the kind of family man who spent a ton of time doing things like yard work or household repairs. He still can't sit around and just relax. He was and is always in pursuit of a new goal or a new challenge.

He's also never been one to love "playing" with the kids. He was always teaching or teasing his daughters, his grandkids, or the athletes he coached. Everything was a lesson.

"He would always play with us, but I do think he'd forget that we were girls," his oldest daughter, Shannon, said. "He'd love to tease a lot. We would watch scary movies, like *Frankenstein* together. He loved to play chess. He loved to pull out teeth – literally. If either me or my sister had a wiggly or loose tooth, he would love to pull it out. We would always hide that we had a loose tooth, or not tell him about it."

When the younger daughter, Erin, was at college at the University of North Texas she wrecked her car. At that point, car wrecks and Erin Ward had a special relationship – they saw each other a lot. Bob Ward was not too happy about that pairing. After this particular wreck, she called home with the bad news. Upon her arrival to the house, there was a note for her that read: "Erin – Turn in your car keys. Buy a bus pass. Signed, your ex-father." Mild sarcasm aside, Ward meant what he said, more for his daughter's safety than anything else. Bob Ward's dysfunctional upbringing was full of so many potential derailing potholes that it could have easily led to Ward's own future family being equally

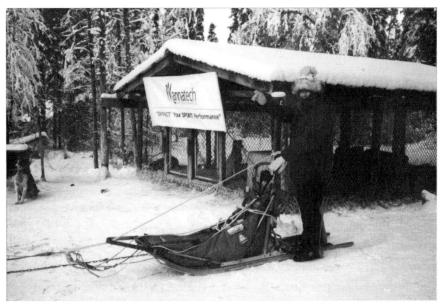

Bob Ward conducting research with sled dogs in Willow, Alaska for Mannatech in the late '90s.

troubled. Fortunately, Ward went 180-degrees away from his own childhood home life to become the provider and stabilizer his father never was.

"Dad was always saying, 'Work, work, work, work, work, work,'" Shannon said. "But I always really looked up to him. He just wanted for us to have it better than he had since he'd no role model at all."

There were two elements in that upbringing that did shape his adult life – the man is completely committed to a life of Christianity. He has always attended church regularly and, in his later years, would often bump into former players at bible school in Dallas. The other was his undying devotion for his wife of more than 50 years, Joyce.

"His commitment to my mother is incredible," Erin said. "He is so devoted to her; the most trouble either me or my sister would ever get in was if we talked back to our mom. He did not want any part of that. She is his world, and family to both of them is everything."

• • • •

As the years began to clip by, the awards started to accumulate and so much of what he did in the '70s and '80s began to come back around. In 1992, Bob Ward was inducted into the Hall of Fame at Whitworth College. In 2003, he was inducted into the USA Strength and Conditioning Coaches Hall of Fame.

A handful of different training revolutions happened between 1990 and the current era, but where most trainers agree is that what Ward was preaching back then – explosion, muscle-based training – is still the best way.

"The reason it's come full circle is that there is no better way," said veteran football trainer Brian Weese, who worked at Texas Tech as a strength coach and now trains future players for the NFL Combine, among other credentials. "The stuff that Bob Ward was teaching back then is the best way. We've had these different crazes and all of that, but at the end it, what he was teaching – the Eastern European/Russian model – is the very best. That's why everybody comes back to it – there is nothing better than what Bob Ward taught."

After Ward left the NFL, the various leagues all began a phase where virtually no one in any sport was not lifting weights. Baseball and hockey players began to look like football players, and basketball players all hit the weights. There were the movements of the "Swiss Ball" phase, then there was an emphasis on cholesterol, and then the term "core training" became chic.

"The bottom line is there is no secret," Vermeil said. "What guys like me and Bob Ward and everybody else figured out is the core is in every exercise."

One of the aspects to strength training that is not so common is there *is* actually such a thing as working out too much. That there comes a point when working out again is pointless.

When a guy like Vermeil played, or even when he was a strength coach at Utah State or Kansas State, if a guy missed a workout it meant he was taking a dive.

Now, through analytics and just common sense, there is so much evidence to suggest that rest will increase future performance. "We had all of these different phases," Dr. Gene Coleman said. "At first, we didn't know what we were doing. Then it was the body-building phase. Then it was the performance phase, which was the Bob Ward phase. Then it shifted to everybody just pump iron and get 'jacked' and get as big we possibly can. And now it's shifted back to what Bob was doing – how can we improve the player's performance?"

• • • •

Today, only the bones of what Dr. Bob Ward brought to the NFL in 1976 remain. It was all "foundational." The NFL is reportedly approaching earnings of nearly $10 billion and is easily the most popular spectator sport in North America. Television ratings for NFL games routinely out-pace all other sports, except college football. In 2014, the third-most watched TV series was Sunday Night Football on NBC. Sports as a whole is a billion-dollar machine.

After more than 30 years at their headquarters in Valley Ranch, the Dallas Cowboys are relocating to a new facility in another Dallas suburb – Frisco. The weight room and exercise areas will all be some variation of what Ward designed for the team in the '80s with updated toys, bells, whistles, comforts, and computers.

The use of computers in sports has grown 100-fold since Ward first increased their integration with the Cowboys. Computers are in cars, in gas stations, and on airplanes. The Internet has changed the world. Instant communication has revolutionized nearly every business, created new ones, and permanently disabled others.

The workout plans he created and invented still exist in their basic form, with a few modifications, except that these workouts are no longer just for the

Dallas Cowboys, the NFL, or pro jocks. Amateur workout junkies now do what Ward had the Cowboys doing. Guys jump on boxes. Sprinting is no longer for Olympic runners. Boxing and MMA are viewed as complete workouts. Sports psychology is a major part of academia and professional franchises.

Bob Ward believed in trying everything because, as a former athlete, he knew one inescapable truth when it comes to sports – if the athlete believes that lifting weights, talking to a sports psychologist, or wearing multi-colored socks is the reason they are performing well, then that is the reason they are performing well. You never know what is going to work until you try it. In a hyper-intense and savagely competitive place like sports, finding those extra 36 inches may ultimately be the difference between winning and losing.

At home, Bob Ward's legacy is his enduring marriage, two daughters, and fleet of grandchildren. He has been in the same home for more than 30 years, and he is surrounded by family and friends, both at church and elsewhere.

Professionally, the man left long and enduring footprints that are routinely stepped in though seldom acknowledged. What Ward believed and implemented would eventually transform the NFL and push it to places it had never previously gone. A part of the NFL – training, preparation, and evaluation – does not look the way it does today without Dr. Bob Ward.

"I really don't think it matters who knows or who did it first, but that it was done," Hall of Fame football coach Mike Ditka said of Ward. "But Bob Ward was the first guy to do it."

EPILOGUE

To be able to write one's life story is something everyone should do for his own family's history. Passing on their experiences, positive, or negative, that could help their families and friends. "Accentuate the Positive and Eliminate the Negative" could be very useful as they weave their own life stories.

Remembering the experiences that were used to weave the tapestry of over 80 years of my life would have been a difficult task for me if I hadn't been taking all the "Brain Power Super Nutrition" over the years. It has been an interesting trip back in time, especially with Mac Engel, my writer. You guessed it; Mac had to be taking my "Brain Power Nutrition" to keep up.

(Mac wasn't – he drank coffee).

The impact of the world circumstances that defined the Greatest Generation during WWI, WWII, and the Depression, influenced my dad and mother as it did many others during that time. They weren't perfect by any means, but they played a big role in keeping America "The Land of The Free and The Home of The Brave." Obviously, it had to have been a big influence on them, and on me, and my brothers, Maurice and Paul, and my sister, Marilyn, during our early years of development.

Every aspect of my career was "Focused on Being the Best You Can Be" with a big emphasis on winning. There isn't any substitute for winning. A review of any world history book will support the role that winning has played from time immemorial. The following quote from the book *Gates of Fire* – historical fiction about the battle at Thermopylae - by Steven Pressfield is a good summary of the consequences of defeat and how important winning was to the Greeks.

"Each man of Greece knew what defeat in war means and knew that sooner or later that bitter broth would complete its circuit of the table and settle at last before his own place."

My WWII experiences as a youngster, along with the influence of sports, played a big part in my career. My life story has been influenced by constantly searching for the "Sine Qua Non," or essential conditions. As

I moved to different careers, I found that these same principles worked in sports, business, and life. All I needed to do was apply them to the specific situations that I was in at the time.

Not many people have had the experiences that I was blessed with before Tom Landry hired me in 1976. It included my time as an athlete, undergraduate, and graduate education, teaching and coaching at the high school and college level, research, USOC Elite men and women's programs, USMC active duty, along with many scientific educational programs, as well as competing as a Masters Athlete.

It has been amazing to see how all of these experiences contributed to my proclivity of being open to a multitude of creative ideas for improvement, but also, in general to the other post "America's Team" applications that I have had in sport, business, and life that followed after my last play in the NFL: 4th-and-1 on the New York Giants' 1 yard line.

Good Luck in *your* Quest on "Becoming The Best *You* Can Be."

– Bob Ward, July 2015

ACKNOWLEDGMENTS

Like any project, there is never just one person that makes its conclusion a possibility. There are two names on the cover of this book, but there are so many others whose time and efforts make it possible.

I am indebted to many individuals and institutions with which God has blessed me throughout my career that have served as guiding lights in helping me search for better ways of improving human performance.

No question as to who heads my list – Joyce, my wife of 59 years. From day one in our marriage to-date, she has been an invaluable emotional and technical storehouse of knowledge. I can't thank her enough for her unending support. Right after Joyce are my daughters, Shannon and Erin and their husbands and families.

A special thanks to my many mentors who opened my eyes with their futuristic vision of human performance based on their personal experiences, and research: Dr. John Cooper, Indiana University; Dr. Jim Counsilman, Indiana University; Dr. Arthur Slater-Hammel, Indiana University; Dr. Paul Ward, Sports Scientist, USOC, Professor, Fitness Industry, Masters Athlete; Dr. Ralph Mann, CompuSport On Field Analysis; Larry Brown, Power Trainer; Dr. Peter Snell, UT Southwestern Medical School; Dr. Jim Stray-Gundersen, Kaatsu; Dr. Larry Gettman Research; Dr. George Kondraske, Human Performance Institute, University of Texas-Arlington.

A huge thanks to Tom Landry, Dallas Cowboys NFL Hall of Fame Head Coach from 1960 to 1988 for hiring me and allowing me the unbelievable freedom to do research and search from coast to coast for scientific ways of identifying "The Perfect Cowboy." In fact, the position was so unique that, by commission and omission, the chances of it being duplicated again are very unlikely.

In 1974 Dan Inosanto, a Whitworth University Football and Track athlete and friend, opened the door to the martial arts, Bruce Lee's Jeet Kune Do (JKD), Filipino Escrima, and many other forms of martial arts for me. Dan trained me in the Martial Arts while I was teaching at Fullerton Community College so we could add Martial Arts and Fencing Courses to our students. I'm grateful to him for opening that door.

And, finally, I would like to give Mac Engel a huge thank you for helping me with *Building the Perfect Star*. It was an arduous journey, I am sure, to sift through the mountain of material I gave him and do the numerous interviews the book contains. It has been my pleasure to have worked with Mac and to get to know him. I appreciate his writing talents and his taking a walk down memory lane with me.

—Bob Ward, 2015

• • • •

Claire Reagan, editor at Ascend Books; I am gracious for her efforts to make this project much better than my original drafts, and for listening to me endlessly pout.

Chris Drummond, Publication Coordinator at Ascend Books; her patience is appreciated.

Bob Snodgrass, Publisher of Ascend Books; thank you for reaching out to me for this project, and patiently listening to me when I whined and moaned about the process.

All of the people who graciously gave me their time to be interviewed for this book: Dr. Jim Stray-Gundersen, Dr. Peter Snell, Dr. Ralph Mann, Alan Carricker, Dr. Paul Ward, Dan Reeves, Roger Staubach, Walter Covert, Charlie Waters, Gene Stallings, Brian Baldinger, Timmy Newsome, Butch Johnson, Bob Breunig, Gil Brandt, Cliff Harris, Tom Tellez, Tom Grieve, Rick Carlisle, Mike Scoscia, Dr. Gene Coleman, Mike Ditka, Kevin Callaway, Brian Weese, Thomas "Hollywood" Henderson, Dave Murphy, Joe Juraszek, Diana Inosanto, Dan Inosanto, Andy Dalton, Travis Frederick, Trumain Carroll, Dr. James Andrews.

A special thank you to Randy White for graciously writing the foreword for this book.

Dallas Cowboys public relations assistants Scott Agulnek and Joe Trahan for allowing me access to files and photos of Dr. Bob Ward during his tenure with the team.

Dallas Mavericks public relations staff members Sarah Melton and Scott Tomlin for assisting me on information history with that franchise.

SMU director of athletic media services Brad Sutton for patiently helping me set up some interviews.

Thank you to my spouse, Jennifer, for prodding me, reading some of the chapters, and for patiently understanding the process that is writing a book. Thank you to our daughter, Vivian, for understanding even though I know you don't just yet.

And mostly, thank you to Bob Ward and his wife Joyce for their considerable efforts, patience, and persistence. This is your story, and it is my sincere hope this book is worthy of a significant, meaningful professional career and life.

— Mac Engel, 2015

ABOUT THE AUTHORS

D̲r. Bob Ward was born on the Fourth of July, the son of a World War I veteran. He came from modest means, even living with his three siblings in a sort of orphanage at the age of six. Ward became a self-made man and one of the most important players in the evolution of professional sports. A former small college All-American, Ward learned by doing. He trained. He played. He coached.

Ward earned his Doctor of Physical Education from Indiana University and studied sports science at its infancy with the U.S. Olympic team. He took that education and went on to implement it with Dallas Cowboys in the mid-70s where he joined Tom Landry's coaching staff as the NFL's first full-time conditioning coach. While activities such as yoga, CrossFit, and martial arts are now common, Ward was already implementing these programs with pro athletes and would revolutionize the way they athletes prepared and trained.

Ward believed in analytics long before it became a part of sports vernacular. His ideas studying and analyzing athletes and movement completely changed the way individuals trained and prepared in sports. What strength and performance coaches, and the athletes themselves, do today to prepare can be traced back to Dr. Bob Ward.

M̲ac Engel is a sports columnist with the Fort Worth *Star-Telegram*. He has written two books: *Tony Romo: America's Next Quarterback* and *Texas Stadium: America's Home Field*. He has covered the Texas Rangers, Dallas Stars, Dallas Mavericks, and Dallas Cowboys as well as multiple Super Bowls, Olympics, NBA Finals, Rose Bowls, and college football championships.

His blog, "The Big Mac Blog," was named the Best Blog in Texas according to the Associated Press in 2012. It finished third in 2014.

Engel has served as an adjunct professor of journalism at TCU Schieffer School of Journalism and currently serves as an on-air personality and contributor to CBS KRLD *The Fan* in Dallas.

BIBLIOGRAPHY

Chapter 1 – You're Fired

Galloway, Randy. "Lengthy Training Camp, preseason games produce one thing: Injuries." *Fort Worth Star-Telegram*. Aug. 17, 2010.

Werder, Ed. "Pumping Iron Tops Priorities: Cowboys' weakness blamed for TD failure." *Fort Worth Star-Telegram*. Dec. 18, 1989.

Chapter 2 – A Difficult Start

Boy Scout Oath: http://www.scouting.org/Home/BoyScouts.aspx

Hyson, Sean and Guarneri, Brandon. "Muscle Paradise! Men's Fitness looks back at Muscle Beach and the golden age of bodybuilding in Venice, Calif." *Men's Fitness*. May 2007.

Chapter 3 – Billion-Dollar Industry

Berman, Zach. "Early Birds: Draft pick signings, changes to training/operations staffs, Connor Barwin's concert." *Philadelphia Inquirer*. May 13, 2015.

Kahn, Jeffrey. "Dallas Cowboys hope virtual reality can better prepare players." *247 Sports*. June 12, 2015.

Chapter 4 – The Long Shot Lands on America's Team

Ghosh, Palash. "Dallas Cowboys and the Indian: How a Computer Statistician From Uttar Pradesh Helped Create 'America's Team.'" *International Business Times*. Oct. 25, 2013.

Durso, Joseph. "Fearless Fosbury Flops to Glory." *The New York Times*. Oct. 20, 1968.

Chapter 5 – Predictions

Ward, Dr. Bob. "Superconditioning Technologies For Sports in the Twenty-first Century." *National Strength and Conditioning Association Journal*. June-July 1982.

Engel, Mac. "The NFL Combine Should Adapt Its Drills and Activities for Football. *www.star-telegram.com*. February 16, 2015.

Chapter 6 – Improving the Dallas Cowboys

Engel, Mac. "Buyers Beware: The case of Terrell Owens reminds teams that take on difficult personalities: It's often more trouble than it's worth." *Fort Worth Star-Telegram*. November 13, 2005.

Chapter 7 – Applying Science to High Performance

Sullivan, Ronald. "Anatoly Tarasov, 76, Innovative Coach of Hockey in Soviet Union." *The New York Times*. June 24, 1995.

Moran, Malcolm. "Cowboys Floating in the '80s." *The New York Times*. May 18, 1981.

Chapter 8 – The Analytic Apostle

Polaroid History: www.polaroid.com

Bresnahan, Mike. "How the Lakers Lost LaMarcus Aldridge." *The Los Angeles Times*. July 2, 2015.

Thomas Jr., Robert McG. "Pro Basketball; Celtics' Lewis Dies After Collapsing in Gym." *The New York Times*. July 28, 1993.

Beck, Howard. "Curry Faces Tests To Evaluate Risk Factor." *The New York Times*. Oct. 5, 2005.

Chapter 9 – Panning for Gold

Engel, Mac. "Buyers Beware The Case of Terrell Owens reminds teams that take on difficult personalities: It's often more trouble than it's worth." *Fort Worth Star-Telegram*. Nov. 13, 2005.

Himmelsbach, Adam. "Years before drafting him, Celtics eyed Marcus Smart." *The Boston Globe*. June 21, 2015.

Chapter 10 – From Martial Arts to the UFC

Sandomir, Richard. "Fox's Glazer Straddles Jobs as N.F.L. Reporter and Trainer." *The New York Times*. May 27, 2010.

Stapleton, Arnie. "NFL Pass Rushers turn to Martial Arts Tactics." *Associated Press*. December 24, 2014.

Chapter 11 – Performance Enhancers: The Good, The Abused & The Illegal

"Sports and Drugs: Historical Timeline." *ProCon.org*. Aug. 8, 2013.

Simers, T.J. "Svare Works to Remain Ahead of his Time." *The Los Angeles Times*. July 31, 1992.

Rutemiller, Brent. "Doping's Darkest Hour; The East German's and the 1976 Montreal Games." *Swimming World Magazine*. Nov. 28, 2013.

Harvey, Randy. "USOC Disavows Ward, Says He Did 'Disservice'" *The Los Angeles Times*. July 3, 1984.

O'Connor, Anahad. "'Fed Up' Asks, Are Calories Equal?" *The New York Times*. May 9, 2014.

Chapter 12 – The Empire Crashes

Wojchiechowski, Gene. "NFL Strike: 1982: A History Lesson Not Learned" *The Los Angeles Times*. Sept. 23, 1987.

Myers, Gary. "Jones Buys Cowboys, fires Landry." *The Dallas Morning News*. Feb. 26, 1989.

Watkins, Calvin and Taylor, Jean-Jacques. "Jerry Jones: Pretty Serious Risk." *ESPN. com*. Feb. 25, 2014.

Chapter 13 – Footprints in the Turf

Boudway, Ira. "The NFL's Secret Finances: A $10 Billion Secret." *Bloomberg.com*. Sept. 4, 2014.

For further information on Dr. Bob Ward's research, please consult *Encyclopedia of Sports Speed* by George B. Dintiman and Robert D. Ward, *Encyclopedia of Weight Training* by Paul E. Ward and Robert D. Ward, and the Sports Science Network at www.sportsscience.com.

Visit www.ascendbooks.com for more great titles!

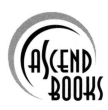